THE TOTAL
PACKAGE

THE TOTAL PACKAGE

How to Create Your Ultimate Lifestyle
and Live the Life of Your Dreams

ANTHONY PALMER

Castiglione Publishing, Inc.
8374 Market Street, Suite 153
Lakewood Ranch, Florida 34202
2004

Printed in the U.S.A.
Second Edition

For more information or to order copies of this book, contact

Castiglione Publishing, Inc.
c/o Bookmasters
30 Amberwood Parkway
Ashland, OH 44805
800-247-6553
Fax: 419-281-6883

Jacket by Phyllis Chotin

ISBN 0-9744453-0-4

www.AnthonyPalmer.net

Dedication

*To my wonderful parents, Anthony and Julia Palmer,
who always believed in me. Your love, encouragement,
and enthusiasm for life serve as the inspiration
for this book. Your positive and uplifting thoughts and
words are appreciated more than I could ever say
and are with me always.*

Acknowledgments

Publishing a book is not a solo project. During the process of creating *The Total Package,* I had the very good fortune to work with a fabulous team of dedicated people. Creating this book has been an incredible experience I'll never forget. However, it would not have been possible without all the wonderful and talented people I had the opportunity to work with.

First, I would like to thank my good friend and collaborator Lillian Griffiths, who was with me from the very beginning, when *The Total Package* was just an idea. Thanks, Lillian, for providing your word-processing expertise and creative ideas as well as much appreciated encouragement. I cannot thank you enough for all you have done. Thanks also to Lillian's sister, Sonja Hough, for providing excellent assistance at an important juncture.

Special thanks to my wonderful photography, lighting, and digital imaging team. I sincerely appreciate your many hours of hard work and dedication to *The Total Package* project. I hope you had as much fun as I did, even though so much work and concentration were involved. Extra special thanks to the exceptional Steven Martine. Steve, thanks so much for making every photography session a wonderful experience! Thanks Mike Mac for your valuable assistance and insight. Thank you Gregory Payne for your wonderfully artistic talents! Thank you, Mike Tompkins, for your special digital imaging talents.

Thanks to Phyllis Chotin and Jewel McKeon, who inspired the design team with their creative imagination and ideas.

Many thanks to my talented and dedicated editor, Judith Pendleton, whose many years of experience helped pull it all together for the design team at a time when we needed her most. I feel very fortunate to have worked with such a true professional. Thanks to Lana Paton, Jeff Rhodes, Sharri Sable, Arlene Eisele, and Maria Smith at Thomson-Shore for the excellent service you provided while printing *The Total Package*. A special thank you to Christina Adcock for your talented efforts, fabulous suggestions concerning housing expenses and nutritional terminology, and particularly for your attention to *every* detail!

My special appreciation goes out to one of the finest physicians in the country, Rebecca Holly Marshall, MD, for all of her expert medical advice regarding both traditional and preventative medicine as well as her help in clarifying issues pertaining to various medical terms, nutritional supplements, and herbal formulations.

Thank you to our beautiful and talented fitness models, Susan DeSantis and Kimberly Atwood. Because of your efforts, the "Building a Better Body" chapter was transformed into a true work of art. You are both spectacular! Special words of appreciation go to Vicki Brown, whose fabulous home gym served as the location of the majority of the fitness photos. Thanks to Bobby Francis and the fine people at Gold's Gym in Stuart. Thank you Joe Hammond, Ed Boone, and Chris Evans at Gold's Gym in Bradenton, Florida.

Thank you to the very talented Meg La Borde at Greenleaf Distributors for your fantastic advice and dedication to *The Total Package* project. Your efforts are greatly appreciated, and it's truly a pleasure knowing you and having you as a valuable member of the team. Thank you Clint Greenleaf for your incredible belief and passion in this project!

Very special thanks to Jay Moyles for being so wise. Thank you, Carin Moyles, for your invaluable suggestion.

To my sisters, Cathy Brown and Amy Leuenberger, and my brother, Paul Palmer, for all their love and support. I'm very fortunate to have such a wonderful family.

Thank you to everyone who helped with the success of *The Total Package!*

Foreword

*"Is there anyone so wise as to learn
by the experience of another?"*
Voltaire

OUR SOCIETY has reached the point where each one of us must begin to take responsibility for our own choices and their outcomes. There is no reason that each individual cannot become more or do more with his or her life. We must each reevaluate the balancing act of work, family, and play. The pressures of the workplace along with its impact on family life must be reassessed. Where are your priorities? Where should they be? How can you begin to change them? Personal physical fitness needs to be recognized as critical to longevity. Not only diet, but physical training and nutritional supplementation are important. Spiritual well-being also plays an important role and must be preserved. We all need hope.

The world is a dynamic place. Today the world is taking on new characteristics that are affecting each one of us. The United States and global economies continue to be harshly impacted by terrorism and regional conflicts, which have the ability to adversely impact us for years to come. Many of the jobs that were lost will probably never be replaced. Instead, employers looking to satisfy stockholders will replace those employees with technology. That technology will require fewer overhead expenses, but it will lack the personal touch. Many displaced employees will be forced to find another avenue by which to support their families. Unfortunately, returning to school for higher training is not always realistic. As a parent, I know that bills must be paid and children need to be nurtured. In many cases, parents will look to a home-based business solution in order to provide for their families. The trend towards home-based business allows parents more opportunities to participate in the upbringing of the children and take more of a hands-on role. This is going to require people to take more control of their destiny and, in many cases, to acquire a more entrepreneurial attitude.

Taking control of your destiny involves more than just a career reassessment. Not only is your career affected by your choice of lifestyle, but so is your health. What you consume every day directly affects your longevity. "You are what you eat" is a very true statement. The American diet is filled with fat and refined carbohydrates. Because of this, the number-one cause of death in the United States is heart disease. A simple decision to eat a more balanced diet can help increase your longevity by decreasing cholesterol/plaque buildup that promotes heart disease and stroke. A balanced diet also results in decreased obesity. As the obesity rate decreases, so will the rate of type 2 diabetes mellitus, which is directly correlated to obesity. Decreasing diabetes mellitus also helps to decrease the risk of heart disease. These few minor changes also decrease the risk of breast cancer and colon cancer—other common killers in the United States.

Regardless of your current diet and exercise regimen, think in terms of continuous improvement. Anthony Palmer shows you the way to a lifetime of personal, fitness, and career improvement in *The Total Package.* A sedentary lifestyle promotes disease states. By increasing your functional capacity, you can improve your quality of life and longevity—both are important to most of us. As you become more aerobic, destructive habits such as smoking and excessive alcohol intake tend to fall by the wayside. Those adverse habits don't mix well with an active lifestyle. As positive lifestyle changes are implemented, longevity increases. This is because the risk of emphysema, lung cancer, heart disease, ulcers, bladder cancer, cirrhosis, esophageal cancer, and gastric cancer decreases.

Nutritional supplements are also important as you make the decision to live a longer, healthier life. Many nutritional supplements have been proven to be protective whereas few prescription drugs are truly protective. Prescription medications may help with symptoms but do not necessarily prevent the progression of disease. Just a few examples of beneficial nutritional supplements: Vitamin E decreases the risk of Alzheimer's disease, heart disease, and fibrocystic breast disease. Folic acid is also cardiovascular (heart) protective. Soy has been shown to decrease the risk of prostate cancer along with decreasing postmenopausal symptoms. B-complex vitamins are also important. Gingko biloba helps with cerebral circulation. Calcium is an important source for bone strength and growth along with Vitamin D and other vitamins. Every day we are learning more about how important it is to maintain a healthy lifestyle, which includes taking good-quality nutritional supplements. If each one of us can make this a part of our daily routine, we can decrease the high costs of health-care in this country and reduce the need to be on expensive prescription medications that can have adverse side effects.

Anthony Palmer has put together a formula for success, custom-designed for today's fast-paced and changing society. His multidimensional work focuses on the fact that all of the parts of an individual's life must function in unison in order for the person to be successful. Achieving one's goals is not an accident. It requires hard, persistent work. One must be "alive and thirsty" in order to pursue ultimate success. Mr. Palmer's book is a proven road map for this lifelong journey. The journey, if followed with passion and honesty, can be most fulfilling. He has carefully integrated business and technology with fitness and good nutrition as a means of achieving health and prosperity. Anthony Palmer's uplifting yet practical success formula has allowed me to expand my thinking and resulted in a more positive and fulfilling lifestyle for myself and my family. In gaining the wisdom Anthony presents in *The Total Package,* you will also experience many positive and long-lasting lifestyle changes.

Life is how you perceive it and what you do with that perception. May yours be blessed and fulfilled.

REBECCA HOLLY MARSHALL, M.D.

NOTICE

This publication is designed to provide accurate and authoritative information regarding the subject matters covered. It is published with the understanding that the publisher and author are not engaged in rendering accounting, legal, medical, or other professional services in this publication. If legal, medical, financial, accounting, or other professional advice is required, the services of a competent professional should be sought. You should consult your doctor before beginning any diet or regimen of exercise. The publisher and author expressly disclaim any responsibility for any liability, loss, injury, or risk, personal or otherwise, which is incurred as a consequence, directly or indirectly, of the use and application of any of the contents of this book.

Contents

Introduction

THERE ARE an estimated 400 billion stars in our own Milky Way Galaxy and over 80 billion galaxies detectable in the universe. In fact, the Hubble Telescope, hovering 380 miles above Planet Earth, has already shown us that the universe is not only limitless but rapidly expanding! Much like the universe, you have the infinite power inside of you to create your ultimate lifestyle, a lifestyle free of limitations or boundaries. From this moment forward, acknowledge that you have the choice, the freedom, and the infinite power to design your life exactly as you want it to be. There are no guarantees that it will be fast or easy; little that is worthwhile in this world comes quickly or easily. We are all bombarded with tempting offers such as "get rich quick," "lose 20 pounds fast," "0% interest credit cards," and "fitness without exercise." It's all part of the fast food and immediate gratification mentality we have long been subjected to by multi-million-dollar Madison Avenue advertising and low-budget hustlers. Creating your ultimate lifestyle is about constructing a life that is *built-to-last*, creating permanent change built on a solid foundation, not on some get-rich-quick or weight-loss scheme advertised on radio, on television, in the newspaper, or on the Internet.

Never underestimate what you can accomplish. To do so would be accepting defeat before you've even gotten started. You are capable of achieving anything you truly desire in all areas of your life. You have the power to decide whether or not you will design the lifestyle you most desire. If you don't, it's a pretty safe bet someone else will design one for you. Adversity is a completely normal part of the journey to your lifestyle of choice, and many decide that giving up is easier than overcoming the obstacles that inevitably crop up along the way. View adversity as a sure sign that you are growing and progressing in a very positive way. It's not the adversity that counts, but what you do with it.

A Balanced Lifestyle Approach

More than a decade ago I began a career as a financial advisor. After starting out at American Express Financial Advisors, I moved on to form my own financial advisory practice in 1995. One day during the summer of 2000, while meeting with a client, I began to realize that our conversation was about a great deal more than just numbers on an investment statement. At this time, I began to realize that I was consulting with this client not only about her investments and financial planning, but about her entire *lifestyle*. I also realized that I was having similar conversations with many of my clients. In addition to the typical discussions about investing and retirement planning, our conversations often included subjects such as career, family, diet, nutritional supplements, fitness programs, real estate, technology, as well as the fast pace of change in society and the world. It was obvious that creating the ultimate lifestyle required much more than a discussion about money. The ultimate lifestyle for my clients required an integrated and balanced approach, with every area of their lives working in harmony with all other areas. What I had realized at that point was that my life experiences and education in the fields of technology, investments, real estate, fitness, nutrition, and positive thinking were allowing me to help clients not only to achieve their financial goals but to also create their ultimate lifestyle.

Make no mistake about it, money is a necessary and valuable commodity. However, contrary to popular belief, being wealthy, in and of itself, will most likely not make you happy. This concept of success is very one-dimensional and shortsighted in nature. The view that money is the complete solution to a happy and fulfilled life doesn't take into consideration that achieving your ultimate lifestyle is not at all about what anyone else thinks is desirable, but is completely about what *you* want and desire most. What is most important is the lifestyle that will provide the most fulfillment and deep-down satisfaction for you. If being wealthy is your goal, that's great, but don't fool yourself into believing that money alone will fulfill all your dreams.

Creating your ultimate lifestyle—the primary theme of *The Total Package*—is about achieving a sense of balance in all areas of your life. *The Total Package* is specially designed to help you create your ultimate lifestyle, whatever you choose it to be. It is based upon creating positive change in key areas of your life including your mental attitude, goal achievement, your home, finances, health, diet, nutritional supplementation, fitness program, career and technology. You will learn, step by step, how to achieve success in all areas of your life.

There has never been a greater opportunity for you to achieve anything you want from life, whatever that may be. Technological innovations—including integration of Internet, cellular phone, TV, and personal computer (PC) technologies—are opening up tremendous new opportunities in all areas of our lives. The idea of living and working anywhere you desire is now both practical and achievable, particularly considering major advancements in technology. Many Americans are choosing to move themselves and their families to smaller towns and new areas of growth, away from the traffic and congestion of cities and suburbs. Custom-designed homes are now available in many locations and are well within the financial reach of many Americans. In addition, the trend towards home-based businesses is booming thanks to fundamental changes in the U.S. and global economies. Greater use of technology by big corporations has automated many tasks previously carried out by humans. The development of affordable technologies for those seeking to start their own businesses is causing unprecedented growth in the number of home-based businesses.

Of course, central to your long-term success is your health. If you don't have your health, nothing else matters. The trends in health care and fitness today are clearly heading towards a preventative health-care approach. The skyrocketing costs of health care, the side effects and expense of prescription medications, and a growing desire to take control of our own health and well-being are leading more people to take a more proactive approach towards their health. Staying healthy includes eating a well-balanced diet, taking the nutritional supplements that will benefit you most, and following a fitness program custom-made to fit your specific body type and metabolism.

What about your finances? Yes, they play an integral part in attaining your ultimate lifestyle. With the vast amount of information currently available and the lightning-fast speed in which world economies and stock markets move today, many investors feel more bewildered than ever. Always remember there is no greater investment you will ever possess than yourself. However, your money and investments must be managed, and your financial goals must be translated into a well-conceived financial plan.

We are living in an incredibly exciting time, and whatever you desire is out there for you. Make the decision to take the necessary steps to live your ultimate lifestyle, the one you've imagined and most desire. Your possibilities are infinite. The power of the universe is within you. Take hold of that enormous power and place it under your control. Go where you really want to go with your life—starting right now!

The Total Package Owner's Manual

THE TOTAL PACKAGE is designed to provide you with everything you will need on the journey to your ultimate lifestyle. Because of its comprehensive nature and scope, *The Total Package* presents a vast amount of important information. In fact, you could look at *The Total Package* as several books combined into one *total package.* The need to purchase individual books on each and every subject has been eliminated. *The Total Package* is specially designed to give you the financial, fitness, nutrition, goal-setting, success principles, home, mortgage, career, technology, and home-based business information you need in one integrated book. In addition, the book is organized in such a way as to provide you with the greatest amount of information in the least amount of time. Therefore, *The Total Package* will not only help you achieve your ultimate lifestyle, but will allow you to do so in the least amount of time.

Because of the comprehensive nature of *The Total Package,* it would be impractical for you to implement all of the various lifestyle changes simultaneously. Instead, I recommend the following steps to maximize your benefits. First, read the book in its entirety. After that, reread the chapter "A Fantastic Voyage." Because it has to do with your mental attitude, success principles, and goal setting, "A Fantastic

Voyage" applies to all the other lifestyle topics in the book. Take notes or underline any information that is particularly significant to your lifestyle success. After carefully following all of the instructions in "A Fantastic Voyage," begin to focus on one specific chapter at a time. For instance, if you are most motivated to improve your fitness level first, you may want to begin with "Building a Better Body," the chapter on total fitness. And since fitness and nutrition are closely connected, rereading "In Search of the Fountain of Youth," the chapter on nutrition and nutritional supplements, could be the next logical step for you. However, if you are most motivated to put your finances or retirement plan in order first, then you can start on either "Investing for Your Future," "On-line Investing," or "Your Retirement Lifestyle"—or you can read all three consecutively. After reading each chapter, take notes and write down your goals for each lifestyle change on index cards. Complete instructions for goal-setting are included in *A Fantastic Voyage.* Do follow the directions carefully.

Keep in mind that your ultimate lifestyle will require a balanced approach in all of the key areas of your life. While it's important to take a methodical, step-by-step approach to achieving your ultimate lifestyle, be certain to read and incorporate all topics that will help you achieve your most desired lifestyle.

By following these simple guidelines, you will get the most benefit from *The Total Package* in the least amount of time, and, most importantly, you'll be well on your way to achieving your ultimate lifestyle.

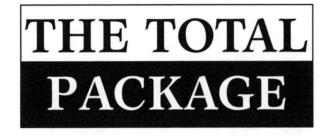

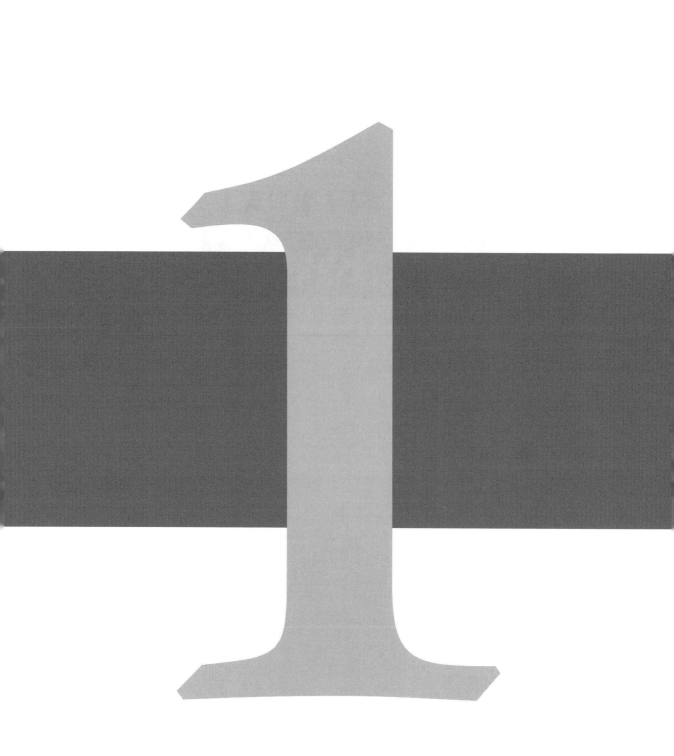

CHAPTER ONE

A Fantastic Voyage

A Fantastic Voyage

**Free your mind and journey to a land of
infinite possibilities!**

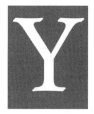ou have at your immediate disposal one of the most powerful forces in the universe. That awesome power is your own thinking. When you acknowledge that truth and begin to use this great power, your life will undergo a magnificent and powerful transformation that will change you forever.

In order to fulfill your life's purpose and achieve your desired lifestyle, you must embark on your own personal "fantastic voyage." Think of this as the most exciting and incredible journey you could ever imagine. The real beauty of this "voyage" is that you possess the total power to choose the destination most attractive and beneficial to you. If it is a truly worthwhile destination you seek, the journey will teach you many valuable and sometimes difficult lessons about life and people. However, reaching your ultimate goal will be a life-changing experience that will take you to the most fabulous and inspiring places conceivable.

In order to achieve a full understanding of how your thinking can change your life, it is of primary importance to understand that you are a unique and complex individual composed of body, mind, and spirit. Your mind, working in concert with your body and spirit, is what will ultimately take you to your goal. Understanding how your mind operates is a critical first step in this process of goal achievement.

Any information processed by your mind will have an effect on your entire being, whether or not you are aware of it, and most of the time you are not. Every word or thought that enters your brain will produce both a physiological (body) and psychological (mind) response. Your mind's past programming as well as your current state of mind will determine your response. You and you alone have the power to respond negatively or positively to the information or thoughts with which you are presented.

Your mind is composed of two different mechanisms: the conscious mind and the subconscious mind. Your conscious mind is the reasoning part of your brain, the part where you make all decisions such as which friends you will have, what home to buy, the right school for your children, etc. On the other hand, there is a second, much dif-ferent and less understood mechanism that your mind employs: the subconscious mind.

—*The Subconscious Mind*—

An extremely important discovery regarding the human mind has been the extent to which our own thinking shapes our entire lives. Your subconscious mind is without question one of the most powerful forces in the universe.

Your subconscious mind has a variety of functions. It controls your heartbeat, digestion, circulation, and breathing. Your subconscious mind controls all of the functions of your body. It never takes a vacation or stops functioning. Your subconscious mind is a protective mechanism that is often interfered with by worry, fear, anxiety, and depression—all caused by the conscious mind. However, the subconscious mind is the controlling mechanism of your mind and, when not interfered with by the negative input of your conscious mind, it will keep all your parts in good working condition. Your natural state is one of harmony unless you start to override your subconscious with consistently negative thoughts originating from your conscious mind.

Your subconscious mind has another wonderful and equally powerful natural function; it can help you achieve whatever you desire in your life. Your subconscious gives you the ability to establish a goal or set of goals that you want to achieve and then will help you get there in the fastest, most efficient manner—if and only if you consistently provide it with the right thoughts and information.

Your mind is goal-seeking by design, much like a radar-guided missile, and will get you to your goal every time if you know how to program it correctly. In essence, your life is really all about achieving goals. Think about it. Getting up in the morning, eating lunch, filling the car with gas, and taking the kids to dancing lessons or baseball practice are all goals! Even though your conscious mind is not fully aware that you are moving in the direction of achieving a goal, your subconscious may be moving you there very quickly. Everything we do in life has to do with achievement, which can be negative as well as positive. For some, their achievements land them in prison; for others, achievements mean personal, professional, and spiritual growth and a life that provides the greatest pleasure and satisfaction. Feeling pleasure does not have to be viewed as a greedy or selfish goal. When you are feeling good about yourself, you are in a much better position to help others achieve their goals as well.

However, whether you choose to achieve positive or negative goals is of no concern to your subconscious mind. It is totally indifferent as to what goals you set. It has no opinion and will not challenge the information you provide it. Your subconscious understands only the information you are providing and will act on this information whether it is constructive or destructive to you or anyone else.

It is also important to realize right now that there are no unimportant thoughts that you can think. Every thought that you have, whether you are consciously aware of it or not, is being recorded on your brain's gray matter, on your own personal computer storage system.

When your brain receives a thought from you, it responds by commanding the release of chemicals into your body and also alerts your central nervous system to any required response or action. If you have ever touched a hot stove or sky-dived for the first time, you know what I am talking about here.

Your subconscious mind will always act upon the thoughts that carry the strongest emotions. Strong, emotional thoughts of the past will continue to determine your direction in life until stronger, more powerful thoughts of the present override them. This is precisely why so many people have problems making positive changes in their lives. When older, more powerful past programming is not overridden by stronger programming in the present, you will feel "stuck in place" and tend to have feelings of hopelessness and despair. You may even feel the urge to give up on your goal because it just seems too difficult and unattainable. Don't dwell on these types of thoughts. Instead, keep moving in a positive and forward direction and these negative thoughts will dissipate. You must replace the old, negative programming of the past with newer and more powerful programming—starting right now! Stronger programming in the present, whether positive or negative, will always replace weaker programming from the past. Having a more positive and fulfilling life is strictly a choice. Your subconscious mind does not care one way or the other whether you succeed or fail in life. The key is to program your subconscious mind with the information and emotions it needs to take you on your journey to your own "Promised Land," the place you want to hold in life, the lifestyle of your dreams. The clock is ticking; the time is now! You can do it! You have all the tools and intelligence you need to achieve whatever goals and dreams you desire. Do not allow yourself to get caught up in the limiting and negative thoughts that most people eventually succumb to. There are a million possible excuses for believing that you cannot achieve something and just as many people out there who are ready to support your erroneous conclusion. Here are some of the more popular excuses:

- I'm too old.
- I don't have the education.
- I'm too tall or too short.
- I don't have the "looks."
- My spouse won't allow me to do it.
- I don't have the money.
- I don't have the time.
- I don't have the energy.
- I simply can't do it.

From this moment forward, believe that you can achieve anything you could ever dream of. Whether you think you can or think you can't, it is up to you to choose how you think. No one else can do it for you. Don't allow anyone else to dissuade you from your intended goal. As Walt Disney once said, "You can achieve anything you desire in this life if you know what you want and how to get it." You can do it and I'm going to show you how right now!

—*The Psychology of Achievement*—

You are successful the moment you take action toward your desired goal.

Why is it that some people consistently succeed with relative ease and others, some of whom are very hard-working and diligent people, consistently fail at achieving their life's goals? The answer is that the unsuccessful people do not have the right "success roadmap" to follow. They are not "programming" their subconscious minds correctly to achieve goals or "hit the target." What I am talking about here is not some mystical or magical technique, but some very practical and relatively simple steps you must be prepared to take to achieve what's important to you. Your future is now. It's time to begin the journey. There's no longer any time to waste thinking about the past, only the fabulous future ahead of you.

—*Five Steps to Success*—

The following five steps to success will take you wherever you want to go in life. This is your life and the clock is running with no time-outs remaining. Let's get started immediately on the road to victory:

Step 1: Infinite Possibilities

"It's kind of fun to do the impossible."
Walt Disney

To successfully arrive at your intended destination(s) in life, you must first change your thinking from one of *limited* and *finite* possibilities to one of *unlimited, infinite* possibilities.

Most people are stuck in a lifelong rut of believing that their potential choices are severely limited. They think in terms of their limited and seemingly comfortable "small world"—their existing home, circle of friends, present occupation, income, vacation schedule, etc. While we should all be grateful for the things we do have, many people get trapped into thinking that this limited world is all that they will ever experience. This finite thinking is merely a mirage or an illusion they have created in their own minds that will ultimately prevent them from achieving their goals. I dare you to even think of the idea of unlimited possibilities and not begin to start feeling better about the future. Think for a moment of the vastness of your possibilities. Go ahead, try it now and feel the exhilaration!

What you must do is release yourself from the bondage of limited thinking and stop thinking in terms of having only one or a few possibilities. You must eliminate that feeling of being stuck or trapped in an illusory world of limited choices you have created in your mind. To experience the awesome power of unlimited thinking, just gaze up at the moon and the stars tonight. Then look beyond them—it's limitless! Isn't this an incredible feeling? Your choices are just as limitless as the universe itself. You must begin to free your thinking to take advantage of the vast and magnificent possibilities at your disposal today.

Step 2: Journey to the Great Unknown

"That which is behind me does not matter."
Ferrucio Lamborghini, founder of Lamborghini Automobiles

Most people get caught in their own self-imposed rut or "comfort zone" and become very comfortable with their existing surroundings and acquaintances. This comfort zone is a very dangerous place to exist, because the greater your comfort level, the greater your reluctance to believe in your unlimited potential and possibilities. Complacency causes you to severely limit your thinking and your available choices. What you know and are familiar with is a result of your past conditioning and what you have been allowing your thoughts to dwell upon. If you have your sights set on a worthwhile goal, it's time to expand your thinking.

What you must do now is free yourself from the rigid mental conditioning of the past and have the confidence and willingness to enter the vast expanses of the great unknown, where the unlimited possibilities and the limitless choices exist. Most people choose the self-imposed prison of past conditioning because it is natural to view something new and different with fear. Fear is the great inhibitor. If you allow it to control your mind and actions, it will keep you stuck in the limited choices of your familiar comfort zone. Chances are, if you are overly comfortable with your existing circumstances, you have fallen into a false sense of security and are currently limiting the number of choices available to you. Free your thinking now so that you can embark on your journey to a more fulfilling life and more attractive lifestyle. Expand your mind and give it the opportunity to take you where you really want to go.

Step 3: Plot Your Course

Dorothy: "But how do I start for Emerald City?"

Glinda, Good Witch of the North: "It's always best to start at the beginning.
And all you do is follow the Yellow Brick Road."
from **The Wizard of Oz**

When you drive in your car, do you normally reach your intended destination? For instance, if you are driving from your home to the supermarket, you would naturally expect to arrive at the supermarket, right? The reason you will arrive at the supermarket and not somewhere else—say the gas station—is that you had a very definite (and familiar) course or road map to follow.

When faced with unfamiliar surroundings and no definite road map to follow, reaching your destination or goal becomes a much different experience. Have you ever gone to an unfamiliar town and tried to navigate around the city without directions or a map? This is precisely what happens when you have no goal to strive for or no road map to follow to your goal. Your mind will not know where to take you, and you will inevitably end up lost. Instead, if you had gotten a map to show you how to reach your destination, you might have made one or two wrong turns, but you would have ultimately reached your intended destination.

Setting goals is really nothing more than choosing the correct "roadmap" to get from where you are to where you want to go. Setting goals is something most people put off to a better time that never comes, or they just never establish them at all. Creating the necessary change and leaving the illusionary false sense of security your mind has created often seems too difficult and painful. If this is the case, it is quite possible that you haven't really identified your real passion in life, or else you are suppressing it because you are afraid you won't be able to achieve it. Without identifying your goals and desires you are setting yourself up to surely fail. Here is what you should do to correctly set your goals:

GOAL SETTING 101: HOW TO ESTABLISH YOUR GOALS

You have infinite power within you
to accomplish any goal you can imagine.

1. *Determine precisely what it is that you desire.* Remember to free your mind and then think in terms of unlimited possibilities. Do not be concerned that your goal seems too difficult or unachievable. Your goal can be anything from buying a new dishwasher to a new Rolls-Royce, from earning a high school diploma to graduating from medical school. Make the goal whatever you wish for: it is yours and yours alone. Your goal will be invaluable to you during times of adversity. It will propel you forward. Think big and do not be concerned about what anyone else will think. Most people are programmed negatively, and they can easily keep you from achieving your goals if you let them. Share your goals only with positive, infinite-possibility-type people. These people are a minority of the population, so be very selective when it comes to sharing your goals.

2. *Next, quantify your goal.* Your subconscious mind needs to know exactly how much money it will take and when you plan to achieve your goal. For instance, your goal may be stated as follows: *"I intend to accumulate $7,500 by July 1st, 2005, in order to take a three-week vacation to the French Riviera and Rome."*

This goal statement includes three crucial elements: a dollar amount, a definite date, and a specific goal. Before he was rich and famous, Jim Carrey, the comedian and movie star, once wrote a check to himself for seven million dollars, an amount he was eventually paid for one of his films. Jim Carrey's check was his goal statement. His check had a dollar amount and a date. The dollar amount was actually the goal itself.

Write your goal statement on one or more index cards and carry them wherever you go. Review your goal statement every morning when you awake and every evening before you go to sleep. This will allow your subconscious to begin thinking of your goal all day, beginning when you first awake, and to dwell on it while you sleep. Remember, your subconscious mind is working even while you are asleep. Say your goal statement out loud and with emotion when possible. The stronger the emotion, the more powerful impact it will have on your subconscious mind.

3. *Determine how you will achieve your goal.* If your present occupation financially limits your ability to achieve your goals, get the training, education, or know-how required to obtain a better paying one. Better yet, start your own business (refer to the chapter on home-based businesses in this book). If you do seek another direction in your life, think about what you really enjoy doing. What is your passion in life? Do you enjoy working with computers, children, animals, real estate, your garden, or investing? If you are going to spend your life doing something, you may as well do what you enjoy. Don't make the mistake of picking a career purely for the money. This is a sure way to buy yourself a lifetime of unhappiness no matter how much money you're making.

4. *Believe in your goals passionately.* You have the power within you to accomplish any goal you can imagine. This is your life, and these are your goals. You deserve the freedom to choose your goals, and you have every right to achieve them. There are many people who will not want to see you achieve your goals because they do not want to see you move ahead of them. Refuse to let anyone hold you back. Pursuing your goals passionately is a basic right that you were born with, and achieving a worthwhile goal is one of the most exciting, exhilarating, and wonderful experiences you will have in your lifetime.

Step 4: Visualize Your Goals

"Everything you can imagine is real."
Pablo Picasso

Athletes and other sports figures teach us a valuable lesson about achieving goals. Golfing great Tiger Woods and tennis ace Jennifer Capriati share one major success principle: they are masters at visualizing success before they even hit their first ball. Great athletes, salespeople, artists, and other professionals know that visualizing the goal before and during the actual effort that takes place to achieve the goal is a crucial component of successful goal achievement.

Visualizing your goal helps program your subconscious mind with a vivid picture of success. Combined with great emotion and passionate feeling, your subconscious will begin to guide you to the successful accomplishment of any goal you desire. Remember that your subconscious cannot tell the difference between something real and something imagined. Unfortunately, most people spend their lives imagining all the negative things that could occur; this ultimately prevents them from achieving worthwhile goals. It's no wonder that the majority of people consistently fail to arrive at their "promised land" in life.

The key to visualizing your desired goal is to vividly imagine yourself "in the present," actually achieving the thing you want the most. For example, if you desire to earn a Ph.D. in psychology, imagine yourself wearing a cap and gown at the graduation ceremonies. Imagine it vividly with passion and affirm your goal statement at the same time. This will send a very powerful message to your subconscious mind. Visualize with passion as you say your goal statement at the same time. Do it in the morning and just before you go to sleep. While you sleep, your subconscious is busy programming your mind. It makes a lot more sense to program for success rather than mediocrity or failure.

**Practice your visualization twice daily and
you will be a step closer to achieving your goals!
Visualization + Passion + Self-Talk = Goal Achievement
When you imagine it, feel passionately about it and say it out loud.
You will achieve it!**

Step 5: Master the Seven Key Principles of Success

*"Go confidently in the direction of your dreams;
live the life you've imagined."*
Henry David Thoreau

During the journey to your most desirable destination you will undoubtedly experience a variety of obstacles—some that you may anticipate, some that you may not. Some of these obstacles may seem to be minor annoyances while others can appear to be downright overwhelming in nature. Make no mistake about it, obstacles will appear. It is part of the natural success-building process to make you earn what you achieve. In addition, there is only one way to meet the obstacles, and that's head on! In order to help you turn your obstacles into opportunities, here are seven key principles of success, which you will want to refer to on an ongoing basis to keep you on track.

THE SEVEN KEY PRINCIPLES OF SUCCESS

Success Principle #1: Overcoming adversity
The greater the adversity, the greater the opportunity.

Just like the early American pioneers crossing the Great Divide, on your fantastic voyage you will encounter some degree of hardship or adversity. In order to deal effectively with adversity, you must begin to view yourself much like a mountain climber ascending to the summit. Mountain climbers experience all types of hardships—some serious, some not so difficult. One day the weather on the mountain may be sunny and pleasant, the next day there may be a blizzard with whiteout conditions. Mountain climbers have to deal with other hardships such as lack of oxygen, frostbite, and avalanches. Compared to the life-threatening conditions experienced by the mountain climber, your challenges will not seem so difficult. However, sharing the same attitudes and mental toughness as the mountain climber will make the difference between success and failure in achieving your goals.

Your ability to withstand adversity, no matter how severe or discouraging, will be a major determinant as to whether you achieve your goals or fall victim to a life of mediocrity and settle for something you really don't want. I encourage you to view adversity as part of your personal growth during your journey. And always keep in mind one natural law of success: the greater the adversity you encounter, the greater your opportunity for success. Embrace adversity; it's a sure sign that you are headed in the right direction.

You must adopt the attitude and conviction to continue moving onward and upward, no matter how slow your progress may seem or how difficult conditions become. As you overcome adversity against all odds and your destination is in sight, you will experience a feeling of exhilaration you may never have felt before. This indescribably fantastic feeling will make overcoming all the adversity worth every bit of energy and effort you put into it—and then some.

YOU ARE DIFFERENT

"If you want to blend in, take the bus."
Slogan of Harley-Davidson Motorcycles

Always keep in your thoughts that, as someone who is committed to overcoming adversity and achieving goals, *you* are going to be different from most people. Most people have no worthwhile goals and therefore limited adversity. Look at yourself as someone who has made the decision to achieve something magnificent and enduring. Being different means that you will experience much greater personal growth than most of those around you, including your family and friends. The humdrum "nine to five" and "TV sit-com watching" lifestyles many lead will begin to seem very boring and pointless to you. In addition, being different will most likely also distance you from those who are not growing in their lives. You will be forced to choose between staying with those who want to stay right where they are or blasting off on your own "fantastic voyage." Don't try to force others to go with you; they must make that decision on their own. On your journey up the mountain you are sure to meet new and exciting "climbers" who share your vision for personal growth. Embrace your individuality, creativity, and motivation. You are truly a unique individual!

Success Principle #2: Become a Master of Change

"Only those who risk going too far can possibly find out
how far they can go."
T. S. Eliot

One thing you can count on in your life is that you will experience change. While this is true, people view and experience change in two very different and opposing ways. The first way people view change is to attempt to prevent, avoid, and limit any changes. Of course, the major reason why most people avoid change is their fear of what that change may bring. The fear of failure, the fear of the unknown, the fear of commitment, the fear of embarrassment and, yes, even the fear of success prevent most people from becoming all they can be. If you've ever been on an airplane that was descending from the clouds and looked down at the residential neighborhoods below, you noticed that most of the houses and developments look extraordinarily similar. Most people find comfort in looking like everyone else, behaving like everyone else, driving the same car, and even living in a house similar to everyone else's. Do not give in to your feelings of conformity. Over the years, I have noticed time and time again that the majority of people are usually heading down the wrong path when it comes to investing their money. People tend to move in herds, succumbing to two of the strongest human emotions—fear and greed. Much the same holds true regarding conformity, which is the opposite of bravery. Do what you believe in and make the changes that make you feel best about yourself. You may be greatly tempted to reverse course at some point in your journey, to go back to the safety and false sense of security of the past. Avoid this temptation at all costs! It can easily keep you from achieving your goal.

A second and substantially more positive way people view change is to embrace and create their own changes. The people who have this philosophy about life are truly in the minority of the population. Creating your own changes means *letting go of your fears*. It's really as simple as that: just let them go! If you are having difficulty letting go of your fears, the best remedy is to begin to take positive actions in spite of them. Your fears are nothing more than an illusion you have created in your own mind. You created the illusion and therefore have the power to transform your fear into desire.

Success Principle #3: Transform Negative Emotions into Positive Energy

"I find that the great thing in this world is not so much where we stand
as in what direction we are moving."
Oliver Wendell Holmes

If you have allowed one or more forms of negative emotions—such as fear, jealousy, depression—to enter your thoughts, do not despair. If you are unhappy with yourself for some reason, feel tremendous guilt over something, fear an upcoming event, or are experiencing any other form of negative emotion, seek to transform your negative energy into positive action. Take positive action in spite of your fears. Emotions can change in a heartbeat. Loneliness can be transformed into love in a split second. Depression and happiness are at opposite ends of the spectrum, but one can move between these feelings almost instantaneously.

Your energy can be used in either negative or positive ways. It is totally up to you how you will direct its power. Always strive to direct your energies toward the accomplishment of your goals. This is actually a very selfless act because your hard work and efforts will lift up and inspire all of those around you. Those who continue to live life with a defeated self-image aren't inspiring anyone, and that includes themselves.

The main thing to remember is to keep changing and growing no matter how things are going. The greater the change you experience, the greater the rewards will be. Do not be concerned with what others think. Most of them will unfortunately be stuck in the same rut they are in now for the rest of their lives. Accept criticism from others as another sign that you are growing and changing for the better. There are many people who do not want you to succeed because of their own defective self-images. View them as victims of their own limited and negative thinking and simply pass them by on your way to an even higher plane of consciousness and achievement.

Embrace change and keep yourself motivated and receptive to change; it is the catalyst that will keep you moving to higher ground on your journey!

Success Principle #4: Perseverance

We have the utmost respect for those who have the courage to persevere.

One of the most powerful tools you possess is that of perseverance, the ability to move forward towards your objectives regardless of adverse conditions. Perseverance is the deep-down feeling that, no matter what happens, no matter how difficult things become, no matter what others say or what obstacles stand in the way, you will arrive successfully at your destination.

It's no wonder that most individuals give up before reaching their goals. After all, this is an era where instant gratification is the desired norm. For most people, persevering through difficult periods to reach their own unique summit in life is simply too difficult and requires too much work. The very temporary satisfaction and tension-relieving act of abandoning the climb to a higher point up the mountain of life is all too easy and tempting.

One evening when I was in high school, a buddy and I were visiting with a very successful executive. The one thing that this person said to us that I remember to this day is "there's plenty of room at the top." I have found that there is, in fact, a great deal of room at the top. It is a place for the courageous few who are willing to do what it takes to reach it. Of course, your definition of the "top" is uniquely your own and should only be what you truly want to achieve.

Your journey will require perseverance—quite possibly a great deal of it. Think of those you know who have had to endure a great deal of adversity but remained persistent and followed through on the attainment of their objectives. Don't you have a great deal of admiration for people like this? Of course you do; we all do. It's why we cheer for the underdogs in an athletic contest; we are pulling for them to succeed because we know that the odds are stacked against them based on our past knowledge of others who have tried. We can relate to the emotions they are experiencing, and we admire their persistence. There are few things one can do that are more likely to gain the universal respect of others than to persist in the attainment of a chosen goal and persevere against all odds. This takes courage, but most people have the ability to be far more courageous than they could ever imagine. We all hold people who persevere in the highest regard, and rightly so. However, perseverance should be a personal accomplishment for you, one that will in turn help improve your self-esteem, self-image, and self-confidence and get you to where you really want to go in life.

There are many wonderful stories of individuals who persevered in the face of adversity and discouragement. Colonel Sanders of Kentucky Fried Chicken fame, after many years of failure finally achieved success at the age of 65. Abraham Lincoln failed at almost everything he tried but went on to become President of the United States. Of course, Thomas Edison, the great inventor, is one of the best examples of perseverance. Edison never considered an experiment a failure, but instead looked at it as one less thing he had to try before he achieved success! When asked why he thought he would achieve results after failing 50,000 times, Edison replied, "Results? Why, I've gotten a lot of results. I know 50,000 things that won't work!" The great Vince Lombardi, legendary coach of the Green Bay Packers, once said, "We didn't lose any games last year, we just ran out of time twice." The art of perseverance is getting up one more time than you have fallen.

Being persistent at something does not mean becoming inflexible. Sometimes you will be faced with an obstacle and it may be in your best interest to find a creative way around it, rather than to continually try an approach that may not be working. Remember, the goal is to create greater happiness for yourself and others, not to "prove" anything to anyone, including yourself. For instance, let's say that your current career is no longer satisfying to you. Well, simply ask yourself what your goal is regarding your career. Is it self-fulfillment, the challenge, or simply the money to allow you to achieve other goals? Switching careers or starting your own home-based business does not necessarily mean you lack perseverance or that you are a quitter. It can simply mean that you have chosen to make a change to another career that is more desirable and beneficial to you. We live in an age where job loyalty has become the exception to the rule. Most employees are caught in a system that encourages cost reduction, often at the expense of employees. Employers are forced by stockholders to cut expenses to the bone, which often means replacing existing workers with cheaper solutions, often technologically based. When workers no longer believe that their employers feel any loyalty towards them, they become more opportunistic about switching jobs, which in turn creates even less loyalty on the part of the employer, and that's how this "vicious cycle" stays in motion. Thus, the trend towards home-based, self-employed workers is one that will continue to grow at a very fast pace. The key thing to remember is to keep your objectives as your reason for persevering. Always act with honesty, integrity, and in a way you would want others to treat you. In other words, follow the Golden Rule: "Do unto others as you would have them do unto you."

Be persistent in your journey. Just keep trying one more time until you finally reach your goal. When you do, you will clearly see how your perseverance played a vital role in your success, and this valuable lesson will help you achieve greater goals in the future.

Success Principle #5: Confidence

*"The only way to discover the limits of the possible
is to go beyond them into the impossible."*
Arthur C. Clarke

Have you ever had the experience of hearing someone speak or just watching some-one walk into a room and thinking to yourself, "That person is very self-confident"? What was it about that person that made you feel that way, and was there really anything that he or she had that you didn't have? The answer is no. You have the power within you at this very moment to be a totally confident person in any way you desire. There is no question whatsoever about your ability to accomplish any-thing you truly want to.

Confidence is the deep-down faith that you are capable of achieving whatever you desire. However, many people harbor false beliefs about themselves that prevent them from feeling confident. What false beliefs are making you less confident than you would like to be? Here are some of the most common false beliefs :

> - I don't have the education.
> - I don't have the money.
> - I am not smart enough.
> - I am not talented enough.
> - I have the wrong genes.
> - I am not attractive enough.

The common denominator of all of these false beliefs is that they ultimately com-pare you to another human being. Comparing yourself to another person is worse than a major waste of time; it ultimately breeds fear, self-destructive habits, and low self-esteem. In addition, comparison naturally creates an inherently negative com-petitive environment, causing those competing to constantly try to "one-up" or "outdo" another person.

From this day forward, begin to think in terms of competing against yourself! Forget about competing against a co-worker, a friend, family member, or even a teammate if you are an athlete. The simple fact of the matter is that you are a completely unique individual with unique talents and abilities. No one on planet earth has exactly these same traits. Therefore, instead of thinking about beating someone else at something, focus constantly on improving what you are doing. A secret that most confident people know is that trying to compete with others actually lowers self-confidence while competing against yourself increases self-confidence and self-esteem. In addition, the habit of self-competition will send very positive messages to your subconscious mind that will help you greatly in achieving your goals. Allow others to help you become better at what you do by learning from them, but always compete against yourself.

Hit your "confidence switch"
and power-up to the next level on the mountain.

Even if you are having difficulty achieving the confidence level you desire at this very moment, simply act as if you are the confident, assertive person you want to be. Think of yourself as acting out the role of a super-confident person until your subconscious mind truly begins believing that you are. In fact, you can use this "act as if" principal in many areas of your life. If you are new at something—say, you are to speak at an important conference or model at a prestigious fashion show—simply do what any good actor would do: act the part until you are comfortable. Just wearing the clothes that help you look the part will take you a long way towards building your confidence and "acting as if." When your subconscious mind takes over with a new image of your new confident self, you will be amazed at how your confidence level skyrockets. Move confidently now, and make your dreams a reality!

Your increased confidence level will allow you to attain heights you never imagined possible. It's time to abandon any remaining self-defeating thoughts you may have about your imagined lack of confidence. Your power to be infinitely confident is ready to be turned on. Why not hit your "confidence switch" and power up to the next level on the mountain? I look forward to meeting you at the top!

Success Principal #6: The Power of Positive Relationships

"Love looks not with the eyes, but with the mind."
Shakespeare

There is one essential ingredient to success that must not be overlooked: the quality of the relationships we form with other people. In your lifetime you will have different types of relationships with different types of people. The relationship we have with our parents and immediate family is usually quite different from the relationships we have with friends and lovers. People come into our lives for different reasons as well. Maybe someone has come into your life specifically to help you through a difficult period, to provide you with physical, emotional, or spiritual support. Whatever the reason, forming positive relationships with others can both help you achieve your goals and bring you happiness on your fantastic voyage.

Of course, one of the great moments in life is finding your soul-mate—someone to share the dreams of the future, to laugh with, to be your best friend, to grow to new levels with you and to share the good times as well as the adversity. You and your soul-mate should complement each other and help each other succeed individually as well as succeeding together with your common goals. Sharing and achieving goals together is one of the great thrills in any relationship. There is certainly nothing wrong with each partner having separate careers, and it can be very healthy for a relationship. However, building dreams together, those great castles in the sky, that's what makes it special! Creating a fabulous lifestyle together is a major personal success, and it's one you can build more successes upon for a very long time.

REACH OUT AND HUG SOMEONE

***Think of someone you'd like to hug and hug that person right now—
you'll both feel wonderful.***

There is tremendous power in simply touching another human being. Touching someone is ten times more powerful than verbal communication. The power of touch can clearly be seen when petting a dog or a cat. It's easy to see the incredible joy they are experiencing! When you give someone a nice hug or a gentle massage, something similar occurs. There is a powerful imprint made upon your mind of that physical encounter. It simply feels awesome, especially when given by someone whom we would like to be touched by. Go ahead, think of someone you'd like to hug and go hug them right now—you'll both feel wonderful!

A new research study by the University of North Carolina–Chapel Hill's School of Medicine suggests that, in addition to making you feel wonderful, hugging may be heart healthy. According to the study, 100 people with long-term lovers or spouses held hands while watching an enjoyable 10-minute video. They then hugged for 20 seconds. Another group of 85 rested without hugging their partners. During the next phase of the study, all participants spoke briefly about a recent event that caused them stress or anger. Memories of negative emotions typically increase blood pressure and heart rates. In the no-hugging group, systolic (upper) blood pressure soared 24 points, more than double that of the hugging group. Heart rates increased ten beats per minute for the no-huggers vs. five beats per minute for the huggers.

Tiffany Fields of the Touch Research Institute at the University of Miami Medical School shows in her research that touching lowers cortisol, a stress hormone. As cortisol is reduced, the body produces serotonin and dopamine, powerful "feel-good" brain chemicals. Extending her study to U.S. and Parisian cafés, Fields concluded that the French touch each other three times more than Americans.

Great relationships have the potential to make our lives infinitely more fulfilling and happy. Select those people with whom you can share a win-win relationship, helping each other to achieve success in all areas of life. These kinds of positive relationships will create a very passionate feeling at some level between you and another human being. I hope you will experience passion of great depth with another human being. It's one of the best feelings you will ever have in your lifetime.

Success Principal #7: Declare Your Independence and Freedom

"Those who would give up essential liberty to purchase a little temporary safety deserve neither liberty nor safety."
Benjamin Franklin, 1759

We in the United States are very fortunate to live in a free society. Acts of terrorism in our country as well as around the world remind us of just how valuable our freedoms are. We live in a society that is based upon a very special document called the Declaration of Independence, signed on July 4th, 1776. I'll never forget July 4th, 1976, the 200th anniversary of the signing of the Declaration of Independence. I was a student attending Northeastern University in Boston, Massachusetts, and was fortunate enough to attend the wonderful July 4th celebration at the Esplanade down by the Charles River. I had no idea what thousands of Americans were about to witness. During the celebration, the great Arthur Fiedler and the Boston Pops Orchestra were playing incredible renditions of fabulous songs like; "You're a Grand Old Flag," "Battle Hymn of the Republic," "The Star Spangled Banner," and the William Tell Overture. The fireworks, the music, the beautiful moonlit evening, and the overflowing masses of patriotic Americans created a wonderfully magical experience that will forever be etched in my mind. It was a very patriotic and proud feeling that everyone that night felt and that, in some way, all Americans share in a unique and special way.

Just as the United States of America has its own Declaration of Independence, from this day forward make your own *personal* Declaration of Independence. You are free on this day to exercise your right to "life, liberty, and the pursuit of happiness." Think in terms of what choices you can make today that will allow you to live your ultimate lifestyle to the fullest. Think without limitations, because your only true imitations are the ones you've created in your own mind. These are some of the freedoms you have today that you should take full advantage of:

- Freedom to live wherever you choose
- Freedom to pursue any career that you wish
- Freedom of speech to tell the world what you think
- Freedom of religion to worship as you please
- Freedom to start your own business
- Freedom to make an unlimited income
- Freedom to attain your educational goals
- Freedom to pursue your health and fitness goals
- Freedom to travel anywhere in the world
- Freedom to break free from limiting or negative people
- Freedom to be happy and have fun
- Freedom to have the family, friends, and relationships you desire
- Freedom to dream magnificent dreams

Start right now by declaring your independence and freedom to pursue the lifestyle that is most attractive to you and makes you feel best about yourself and what you are about to accomplish. Create a win-win experience for everyone. However, beware of those who may try to steal your dreams. *Dream stealers* are all too common in this world. Never let anyone steal your dreams, no matter how hard they try. After all, the freedom to dream is one of the most important God-given freedoms you possess. Declare your personal independence and freedom at this very moment!

—*Your Fantastic Voyage*—

It is my sincere desire that *your* fantastic voyage be filled with ambitious goals, great expectations, a true passion for life, uplifting win-win relationships, and powerful personal growth. Dream big dreams and strive to break free of societal and self-imposed limitations. Let your confidence soar and refuse to be discouraged by anyone or anything. Embark upon your fantastic voyage with "infinite possibility" thinking, in which the only true limitations are those you choose to accept. Make every day a new adventure filled with fresh and innovative ideas. Embrace change, because it will allow you to reach greater heights up the mountain. Celebrate to the fullest all the freedoms that you have. There is no time to waste! Set sail on your fantastic voyage right now, at this very moment. And remember, always follow your heart and have a great deal of fun along the way!

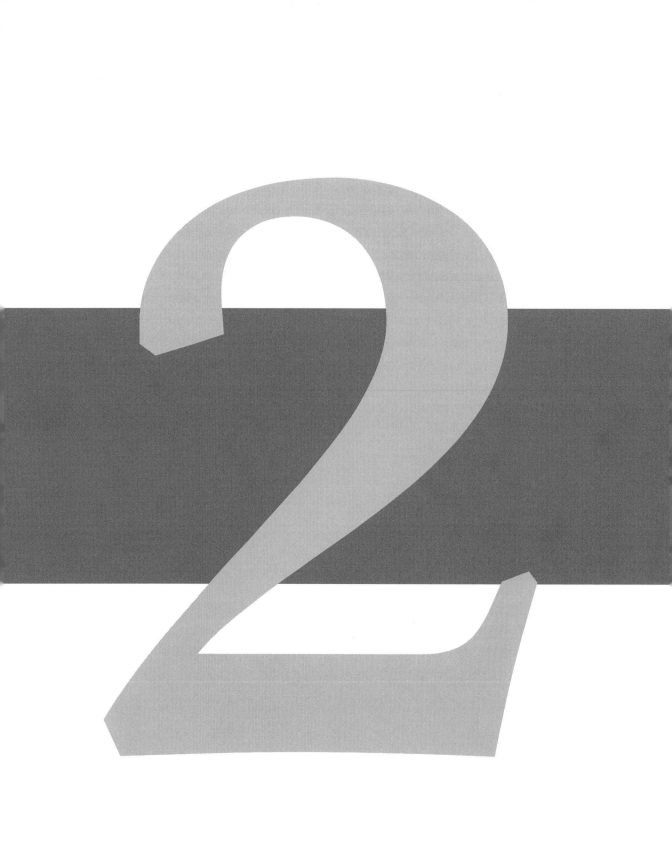

CHAPTER TWO

Home Ownership in the Digital Age

Home Ownership in the Digital Age

The opportunity to live your desired lifestyle wherever you choose has never been greater.

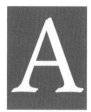

A big part of achieving and experiencing your ideal lifestyle is enjoying that place you call home. A home gives us many emotional, practical, and financial benefits, but maybe the most attractive and pleasurable feature of home ownership is the sense of security, independence, and peace of mind that comes with knowing that we own something of substance that can be shared with our family and friends. A home becomes a special haven, even a magical place to be "home for the holidays," to raise a family, to entertain guests with delicious home-cooking, to relax in the jacuzzi, enjoy the fireplace, or engage in any number of pleasurable activities that provide enjoyment for ourselves and others.

The trends we are experiencing today with regard to home ownership reflect major long-term shifts in the values and desires of today's homeowner. Some of the major factors currently influencing home ownership trends include:

- An diverse population that desires better and more "flexible" lifestyle amenities, including customized home layouts and features

- Interest in homes that take advantage of and blend in with the natural environment

- A shift towards more home-based businesses, which is revolutionizing home designs and creating a long-term trend to comfortably accommodate both home office and family activities

- More time spent in the home due to improvements in home entertainment technologies as well as less inclination to travel, partly because of safety concerns and traffic congestion

- The desire for a more fulfilling and affordable lifestyle with more of a "small town" feeling, including interaction with neighbors we know and a rebirth of community spirit

- Better communication and technology in the form of wireless devices, cellular phones, more powerful and less expensive computers, the Internet, e-mail, personal digital assistants (PDAs), and video conferencing

- Major trend towards home-based on-line shopping and purchasing from "e-tailers" as well as from traditional TV home shopping channels and "infomercials"

—Tax Benefits of Home Ownership—

The fabulous tax benefits offered by home ownership are a major contributor to current home ownership trends. There are few investments that offer the type of tax incentives that home ownership does. And the tax incentives associated with home ownership offer you one overwhelming advantage over other investments offering tax breaks—you can live in this one. Some of the key tax benefits associated with home ownership include:

- Mortgage interest deduction, including up to one million dollars in mortgages secured by a first or second home (such as a vacation home)

- Deduction of points (prepaid interest) at closing. Buyer can also deduct the portion of the property taxes already paid by the seller as a closing cost.

- Real estate tax deduction

- Home office deductions

- $500,000 capital gains income tax exclusion for married couples filing jointly and $250,000 for single people on the sale of your home. (You must have lived in the home for two of the past five years.)

- Deductible interest on home equity loans, up to $100,000

- Deduction of home improvements for health reasons

- Moving cost deductions

- Deductions for land-lease payments as long as the lease is for a minimum of 15 years and isn't associated with land in a trailer park.

Having the best of both worlds is what many of us desire today: the feeling of belonging to a community that reflects our individuality plus our desire to successfully continue our professional pursuits. It's a wonderful feeling to have these kinds of choices available. The opportunity to live anywhere you choose while pursuing your career and lifestyle goals has never been greater. Ultimately, the choice of what type of home you live in and where you live is up to you and reflects your individuality, taste, and lifestyle preferences. Wherever you may find it, there really is no place like home.

—*The Seven Steps to Buying Your Dream Home*—

At first, the thought of purchasing the home of your dreams may seem to be an overwhelming project. Back in the 1950s and 1960s, as in the days of TV's "Father Knows Best," it was the "man of the house" who took care of the financial aspects of the home purchase. Times have changed; more and more single women are purchasing their own homes, particularly as the divorce rate has skyrocketed in recent years. Purchasing the home you desire does not need to be a daunting or unpleasant experience. Think of it instead as part of your fabulous journey, with the chance to live in your dream home as the ultimate destination.

Let's take a look at the seven steps to buying your dream home. Where do you begin your quest for the home that will give you the most home for the least amount of money? The first step begins with you.

Step 1: Identifying Your Ideal Home and Location

The first step in the home-buying process is to ask yourself the following questions, designed to help you identify the type of home you will feel most comfortable about purchasing:

- What type of architecture or style do I prefer?

- What size of home do I want?

- What arrangement do I prefer—a ranch-style, or perhaps a two-story home?

- Do I prefer the newer communities offering "small town" charm and a reflection of individuality, or the traditional suburbs with cookie-cutter homes, or the sophistication of the city?

- Do I want to buy an existing home or have one custom-built?

- How many bedrooms and bathrooms do I need?

- Will I be working from a home office; if so, how will this impact the overall needs of the family?

- What size garage is best for me?

- Is a large kitchen important, or do I want a big deck outside (or both)?

- Do I want a big lawn and pool, or is low maintenance preferable?

- Where would I live if I could choose to live anywhere in the world?

The answer you are looking for here is precisely what are the most desirable home locations and characteristics for you. By identifying these attributes as your first step, you will save a great deal of time later in the process. Choose to live the life you've imagined.

Major advancements in technology, communications, and affordable customized home designs allow you today more than ever before to live the lifestyle you choose, anywhere you want to. Many new communities have been developed with superior planning and infrastructure that are safer for families and that will allow people to select the lifestyle that best suits their needs. In addition, you can do the work that you love just as well in your new location; and with new advances in communication and information technologies, the home-based business concept is more convenient, affordable, and potentially lucrative than ever before.

CUSTOM-DESIGN YOUR NEW HOME

Remember what it was like to have to rely on a real estate professional or an architect to painstakingly make changes every time you wanted alter your new home's floor plan? While professional assistance is certainly helpful, making changes to floor plans has become much simpler; now it's something you can do yourself!

Increasingly, home builders are capitalizing on the power of Internet technologies to allow buyers the ability to quickly and easily custom design their own homes on the Internet. For instance, the custom home builder Toll Brothers (TollBrothers.com) allows you to customize your choice of 55 different model homes available in 22 states across America to your lifestyle specifications. You can choose from more than 450 customizable options for your new home. Some of the options and choices available include standard or "culinary" kitchens, four different types of garages, expanded breakfast areas with "greenhouse" or "bay window" effects, in-law suites, and eight choices of additional rooms depending upon whether you want a home theater, game room, home gym, or a home office. The site allows you to interactively change floor plans as well as print them with ease. You can even take a 360-degree panoramic tour of the home designs and floor plans available.

More and more home builders will be introducing Web sites similar to the Toll Brothers site that will allow you to quickly, easily, and cost-effectively custom-design the home that will best suit the lifestyle needs of you and your family. Even if you decide to hire a professional to help you with your new home's design, the ability to get some idea of the options available and to work with those changes yourself will help you to ultimately make better and more informed home design decisions.

WIRELESS SMART HOMES

It seems like yesterday that home builders were advocating "pre-wiring" homes to make them "technology-ready." While pre-wiring a home may still make sense for some, this "wired" technology is quickly becoming obsolete for many homeowners. A new technology called Wi-Fi (wireless fidelity) allows computer manufacturers to create wireless devices that communicate together. The use of this technology is spreading quickly among homeowners because Wi-Fi allows you to connect all your homes PCs and laptops to a local area network (LAN) or to a high-speed Internet connection without pulling cables through the walls and floors of your home. Also, there's no longer a need to manage all of those thick black cables that created an eyesore and had to be stuffed behind the computer furniture.

To set up a Wi-Fi Internet connection in your home you will need DSL or cable modem service in addition to a small box called a wireless router or access point, which connects all of the devices together. Your computer will also need a wireless interface card. If you have an older computer, make sure that its technology will support Wi-Fi. If you will be using new computers, today all reputable computer manufacturers offer "Wi-Fi ready" computers. Computers with Intel's Centrino microchip technology have Wi-Fi functionality built in, but computer manufacturers such as Dell, Toshiba, and IBM plan to offer consumers additional choices when it comes to wireless chip technology. With this type of set-up you can connect all your home computer devices within 300 feet of one another (the length of an American football field). Besides speed, another advantage of Wi-Fi is that it's inexpensive. For example, Microsoft offers a complete home-based Wi-Fi solution for under $200. If you are still bent on having your entire home network or part of it hardwired, there is a technology called Powerline that allows your network to piggyback on your home's low-tech electrical system. This solution avoids the necessity of having your home wired exclusively for technology.

The applications to support the growing demand for wireless technology are vast and expanding rapidly. Here are some home technologies that are producing tremendous demand for wireless home networks:

- Computer-controlled devices including security alarm systems, security cameras (theft protection and child safety), lighting, music, garage doors, thermostats, and even pool cleaners and heaters

- Home entertainment systems, including home theaters, game systems (Sony Playstation, Microsoft Xbox, etc.), satellite and cable TV

- Support for wireless high-speed Internet connections, such as DSL and cable-modem technologies

- A wireless network connecting all your home PCs, regardless of where they are located in the house. This will save you a good deal of money, particularly if your family has multiple PCs. Your home PC network can be used as the central data center for all of your wireless mobile devices. Information from wireless devices such as cellular phones, PDAs, wireless Internet devices, laptop computers, pocket PCs, and "communicators" (cell phone, PDA, and Internet device in one) can be synchronized with your networked home PC system and stored there as well.

- Video-on-demand, which allows you to watch whatever you want whenever you want

- Interactive TV, a major developing trend that combines the Internet, the personal computer (PC), and TV. With interactive TV, your kids will be able to play computer games with their friends or solve a math problem with a teacher across the street or across the country. You'll be able to switch back and forth between your PC, the Internet, and your TV with a remote control, in addition to having complete personal digital assistant (PDA) capabilities. In other words, you can shop on-line, send an e-mail or instant message to a friend, look up your cousin's phone number, watch Seinfeld or Friends reruns, and write a letter on your PC—all at the same time. The beauty of Wi-Fi, is that you will be able to do all this from the comfort of your living room couch or even poolside while enjoying the jacuzzi!

Of course, let's not forget Grandma and Grandpa, who can easily use inexpensive Internet cameras and voice technologies to see and talk with their grandchildren on the computer screen whether they are down the block or across the country.

The major benefits of a wireless home network will ultimately be realized in the enjoyment, education, fun, and togetherness that you and your family experience from this amazing new technology!

LOCATE YOUR NEW HOME

Look at your quest to find a new home as a magnificent journey filled with great excitement as well as many wonderful learning experiences. In this wonderful world of technology you don't even have to get out of your easy chair to start. In fact, I recommend that you don't! A great place to embark on your journey is at a Web site called BestPlaces.net, which offers a vast amount of information about real estate locations and lifestyle choices throughout the United States and around the globe. Here are some of the great features included in this Web site:

- Profiles and comparisons of more than 3,000 cities using 100 different categories

- Powerful tools to help you find your most ideal place to live

- Examination of over 16,000 U.S. school districts

- Cost of living and salary calculator

- Crime rate comparisons of over 2,500 U.S. cities

- Climate profiles for 2,000 cities worldwide

Another good site to explore when researching new locations is Digitalcity.com, where you can find information on career opportunities, real estate, shopping, travel, dining, and entertainment for major metropolitan areas nationwide.

There is no longer any reason to feel stuck in a location that is unsafe or in any way undesirable to you. For instance, do you love the mountains or is a life by beautiful beaches more to your liking? How does the thought of living near Vail, Colorado, or Hilton Head, South Carolina, sound to you? These are just two of many potential locations; you should not feel constrained any longer. A home-based business venture, utilizing very common technologies, offers you freedoms that could only be dreamed of a few years ago. Your opportunity to live the lifestyle you desire in the location of your choice has never been greater! Of course, this is a decision that will require a great deal of thought, but exploring the possibilities can be a fabulous learning experience and wonderful adventure as well!

Step 2: Determining How Much You Can Afford

You now have a good general idea of the type of home you desire. However, before you call a realtor or explore the Internet to locate your dream home, it is crucial that you first examine your home purchase in terms of your financial condition. The answer to "How much home can I afford?" lies in two underlying questions:

- How much of a mortgage loan can I afford?
- How much can I offer as a down payment?

In order to come up with good solid answers to these questions, it's necessary to get into the general subject of mortgages, the focus of our next step in the quest for your ideal home.

Step 3: Exploring Mortgage Loans

Obtaining a home mortgage today is much easier than it was even a few years ago. However, the mortgage industry today has a much wider variety of choices; consequently, a little more thought has to go into your mortgage selection analysis. Let's go through some fundamentals and move through the mortgage selection process.

MORTGAGE BASICS

Most people do not have $100,000, $250,000, or $500,000 in cash available for a home purchase. Even if they did, most would choose to borrow at least part of the money required. This type of borrowing is called a mortgage loan. There are many different types of mortgage loans. Here are the most common types:

Monthly Mortgage Payment Calculator

30-year Monthly Mortgage Payments

Rate	$100K	$150K	$200K	$250K	$300K
5.0%	$535	802	1069	1336	1604
5.5%	$565	848	1131	1413	1696
6.0%	$597	895	1193	1491	1790
6.5%	$632	948	1264	1580	1896
7.0%	$665	992	1331	1663	1996

15-Year Monthly Mortgage Payments

Rate	$100K	$150K	$200K	$250K	$300K
5.0%	$788	1181	1575	1969	2363
5.5%	$813	1220	1627	2033	2440
6.0%	$840	1259	1679	2099	2519
6.5%	$871	1307	1742	2178	2613
7.0%	$899	1348	1798	2247	2696

30-Year Fixed-Rate

This is the most common type of mortgage loan. The advantages of a 30-year fixed-rate mortgage is that it's the easiest fixed mortgage to qualify for. It does an excellent job of helping you keep your mortgage payments at a minimum; plus you are able to deduct all interest for tax purposes. On a mortgage carrying $1,000 per month in interest payments, you get a $12,000 per year deduction from your gross income. Another advantage of a fixed-rate mortgage is predictability. You know exactly what your mortgage payment is going to be. Most 30-year mortgages allow you to pay off the principal balance of the mortgage (pre-payment), thereby reducing the number of years you will have your mortgage.

15-Year Fixed-Rate

The primary advantage of a 15-year mortgage over a 30-year period is a lower interest rate. This shorter-term mortgage will allow you to pay off your mortgage more quickly, thus building equity in your home faster. The downside to a 15-year mortgage is that your monthly payments will be higher, plus you will be deducting less interest from your gross income than you would with a 30-year fixed-rate mortgage.

The Mortgage Calculator on page 46 will tell you what your monthly principal and interest payments would be on a 30-year and a 15-year fixed-rate mortgages.

For instance, if your 15-year fixed-rate mortgage is $150,000, at an interest rate of 7% your monthly payments are $1348/month. Of course, you will have to include real estate taxes, private mortgage insurance (PMI), and homeowner's insurance to these figures to complete the picture.

30-Year versus 15-Year Fixed-Rate Mortgage: The argument between advantages of a 15-year fixed- rate mortgage a 30-year fixed-rate mortgage has been going on since those two mortgages were invented. As an example, on a $200,000 30-year mortgage, your monthly principal and interest payments at a 7% rate would be $1,331 per month. On a 15-year mortgage, estimate that the interest rate will be about ½% lower than with a 30-year rate. So, at a 6.5% rate, your 15-year mortgage would cost $1,742 per month. An extra $411 per month is a big difference for most people and the primary reason most choose the 30-year alternative; the second is the additional tax savings from the additional mortgage interest deduction.

Adjustable Rate Mortgage (ARM)

With an adjustable rate mortgage, your interest rate will fluctuate along with changing market and interest rate conditions. When mortgage rates go up, your rate will go up. When rates go down, your rate will go down. The major advantage of an Adjustable Rate Mortgage (ARM) is a low initial "teaser" rate. The primary drawback is that your monthly payments may increase when rates head up. However, ARMs have two different "caps" or limits on how high your rate can go. One cap sets a limit (usually about 2%) on how much your rate can go up during each adjustment period (usually once or twice a year). The second cap (lifetime cap) sets the maximum possible interest rate over the life of the loan, which is typically around 6% above the original loan rate.

During times of high interest rates, ARM loans make the most sense because the initial rate is substantially below the rate of a fixed-rate mortgage. During times of lower interest rates, ARMs may make less sense because the difference between the ARM rate and the fixed rate narrows and the rate "spread" is no longer as attractive.

During high-interest rate periods such as the 1970s and 1980s, ARM loans were very popular. During the lower interest rate periods of the late 1990s and early 2000s, however, ARM loans became less desirable than fixed-rate mortgages.

Hybrid Adjustable Rate Mortgage

Hybrid Adjustable Rate Mortgages are a cross between a fixed-rate mortgage and an Adjustable Rate Mortgage (ARM). One example of a Hybrid ARM is the Federal National Mortgage Association's two-step mortgage. This type of mortgage is based on a 30-year payment schedule and is fixed for the first five or seven years, depending on which plan you choose (step 1); then it adjusts only once (step 2). The initial interest rate on these mortgages is typically less than what you would get on a 30-year fixed rate mortgage. After the adjustment takes place, the mortgage remains fixed for the remainder of the 30-year mortgage term. The new step 2 rate has a maximum cap of six percent over the step 1 rate. Other variations of this type of hybrid mortgage will have a fixed rate for either a 3-, 5-, or 7-year period and then adjust annually after the initial term is over.

Hybrid mortgages tend to make the most sense for home owners who plan to sell their homes or pay off the mortgages in full before the initial fixed term is completed. The gamble with a hybrid mortgage is that if rates rise substantially (as they did in the early 1980s), you could be stuck with a shockingly high mortgage payment. For instance, if your initial rate on a hybrid mortgage were 7% and mortgage rates skyrocketed, you could conceivably end up with an interest rate of 13%. On a $200,000 mortgage, you would find yourself paying an additional $881 per month ($2212-$1331 = $881). Ouch!

Another example of a hybrid is a balloon mortgage with lower fixed payments for an initial period, usually based on a 3- to 10-year time span. After the initial period, the entire balance of the loan is due. However, some balloon mortgages allow you to convert to a fixed- or adjustable-rate mortgage after the initial period. With all of the great mortgage alternatives available today, I would suggest exploring fixed-rate and other forms of hybrid loans before seriously considering a balloon mortgage. It's conceivable that the balloon payment could come due when mortgage rates are high, leaving you with little in the way of favorable alternatives.

Government Loans

Agencies of the federal government issue primarily three types of loans:

FHA Loans: Federal Housing Administration (FHA) loans have as their primary benefit a very low down payment, typically 3% to 5% of the purchase price. FHA mortgages have a loan limit that varies depending on the average cost of housing in a given area.

RHS Loans: The Rural Housing Service (RHS), a branch of the U.S. Department of Agriculture, offers low-interest loans with no down payment to low- and moderate-income persons living in rural areas or small towns.

VA Loans: Veterans Administration loans are offered by the U.S. Department of Veteran Affairs. You must be a qualified U.S. veteran to obtain a VA loan. The VA guarantee allows qualified veterans to buy a home costing up to $203,000.

Federal National Mortgage Association Loans

This agency, commonly known as "Fannie Mae," was created by Congress in 1938 to help the housing market during the Great Depression; in 1968 it became a privately held shareholder-owned company. If you have ever shopped for a mortgage, you have probably heard the name. Fannie Mae doesn't actually lend mortgage money directly to home buyers; rather, it purchases and sells residential mortgages in the secondary market through banks. The banks then lend you the money directly. The Federal Home Loan Mortgage Corporation (Freddie Mac) operates in a similar fashion to Fannie Mae. Fannie Mae and Freddie Mac are known for offering low- or no-down-payment mortgages to qualifying individuals with good credit and good income. The Government National Mortgage association (Ginnie Mae) does not actually buy and sell mortgages through banks but helps to insure the availability of mortgages through mortgage-backed securities—investments similar to bonds but carrying the guarantee of the full faith and credit of the U.S. government.

Biweekly Payments: Faster Mortgage Payoff

Here's a simple and effective option. Instead of making your regular monthly mortgage payments: pay one-half the amount every other week. Thus, you'll make 26 half-payments, which is the equivalent of 13 monthly payments per year. A typical 30-year biweekly loan will be paid off in 18 to 20 years; a 15-year biweekly loan would be paid off in about eight years.

Some lenders offer a lower rate on a biweekly mortgage and most require having the payments automatically deducted from a checking or savings account. However, if you have the financial discipline and willpower, you can accomplish the same goals: saving interest, building equity faster and shortening the term simply by prepaying the mortgage. Always check with your mortgage lender whenever making advanced payments on your mortgage. Some mortgage lenders have prepayment penalties that borrowers may not be aware of.

Step 4: Making a Down Payment

Now that you've got a good, basic idea of the types of mortgages available, there is still one more thing to do before you can determine how much home you can afford. You must determine your down payment. The traditional school of thought concerning down payments was 20% of the purchase price. However, the mortgage business has never been more competitive with traditional lenders such as banks and mortgage brokers forced to compete with the up-and-coming Internet mortgage lenders. Because of this, there has never been a better time to obtain a mortgage *and* a favorable down payment. Many home buyers should be able to qualify for a good mortgage rate with a down payment substantially less than 20%. Many will be able to qualify with a 5% down payment or possibly even less. For most people, I would recommend a minimal down payment with the remainder of available funds used to pay off credit cards or build your retirement savings. For our purposes, in Step 5 I am going to use a middle-of-the-road down-payment of 10%.

Step 5: Determining Your Mortgage Payment

Now that you have a grasp of mortgage and down payment basics, let's calculate your monthly mortgage payment to see how much home you can afford. You can plug in any home purchase price you like. I suggest you experiment with a few different figures. To calculate your mortgage payment, use the Mortgage Calculator provided on page 46. Choose a home price and interest rate you believe are reasonable for your circumstances. Remember to deduct your hypothetical down payment of 10% before determining your mortgage amount. For instance, if you are looking at a home purchase price of $200,000 and your down payment is 10%, that's a $20,000 down payment. You would then be basing your mortgage payment calculations on a mortgage amount of $180,000 ($200,000-$20,000 = $180,000). On page 52 you will find a worksheet to help you figure your mortgage payment.

Once you have determined your monthly payments for your new home, you will want to get a good idea of whether the bank will lend you the amount of money you are looking for. In general, the bank will allow you up to 36% of your gross income for housing expenses. To be conservative (banks are conservative, right?) I'll use 30%. Let's say that your total gross income is $60,000 and the bank will allow you

30% for your housing expenses. That comes to $18,000 per year or $1,500 per month. You can use this number to get some idea of what mortgage amount the bank will loan you (after subtracting out expenses not mortgage related). Another avenue to explore when doing mortgage calculations is to go online to Quicken.Com or Lendingtree.com. These sites provide easy-to-use mortgage calculators.

MORTGAGE AND HOME PAYMENT WORKSHEET

30-year or 15-year fixed-rate mortgage payment
based on the Mortgage Calculator .... $_____

Monthly homeowner's insurance .... $_____

Monthly property taxes (based on a percentage
of sales price set by property appraiser in your area) .... $_____

PMI (private mortgage insurance)
(mortgage amount x .006/12) .... $_____

Total monthly home payment .... $_____

In addition to the expenses related to your mortgage, insurance, property taxes, and PMI, you should also factor in expenses such as utilities (water, gas, electricity, phone, cable, high-speed computer connection, etc.), security services, home cleaning, yard and pool maintenance, pest control, homeowner's dues, and any other expenses you will incur. That way you will have a more complete understanding of—and be better prepared to determine—your total cost of home ownership.

Step 6: Let's Go Shopping

Now that you've determined what home price you can afford, it's time to go shopping for two major items: your home *and* your mortgage. Let's start with looking for your new home.

The evolution of the Internet has made the process of buying a home a much different experience from what it was even a few years ago. If you know how to use the World Wide Web to your full advantage, you can become a much more educated and "real estate worthy" homebuyer. After all, the Internet is really about information— in this case, about a tremendous amount of useful real estate information.

THE INTERNET HOME-SHOPPING EXPERIENCE

The Internet is dramatically altering the process of searching for a home. In fact, this process is quickly becoming an entirely new and very exciting experience. On-line search capabilities are continually improving, providing more content, greater ease-of-use, and more freedom of choice when it comes to property selection. After all, the home-buying experience is really about using information resources that will most quickly help you find your ideal home at the best price. The Internet can empower you to choose how much help, if any, you want from a real estate professional (realtor).

Now more than ever before, the Internet allows you, the home-buying consumer, to choose how much of your home search to do on your own. One of the primary reasons consumers are benefiting is that the Multiple Listing Services (MLS) home real estate listings, formerly controlled exclusively by professional realtors and the National Association of Realtors (NAR), are now gradually becoming available to the general public. Historically, real estate listings have been the bread and butter of the real estate industry, and the realtors who controlled the listings essentially controlled the real estate market. While this system remains the status quo in the real estate business today, we are seeing more and more MLS listings opening up to the public. Expanded usage of the Internet is the primary reason for the loosening of the grip on the MLS system.

Regardless of how much help you will or will not want from a real estate professional, there are three Web sites that are a good starting point for your home search:

- Homeadvisor.com (owned by Microsoft)
- Realtor.com (official site of the NAR)
- Homestore.com

While these Web sites are a great place to begin your search, keep in mind that they all have agreements with realtors and a major goal of obtaining valuable real estate listings. Even with the obvious bias towards the seller's point of view and the objective of producing real estate commissions, these sites can help you get a good idea of what homes are available in your location and in your price range.

Virtually all of the real estate Web sites let you search for homes by location or zip code; then you can narrow the search by supplying a price range and detailed home preference information. For example, Realtor.com has the largest on-line database of homes for sale—currently, about 1.5 million. Realtor.com also has a "find a neighborhood" section that can help you identify desirable communities if you are moving to a new, unfamiliar neighborhood. This site can also take you on a 360-degree virtual video "tour of homes." These tours make you feel as if you are standing in the center of a room and let you look around by clicking your computer's mouse.

A useful site for home-sellers seeking a real estate agent is Homegain.com. This site asks sellers to describe their homes anonymously and provide an expected asking price. Local agents then submit proposals to win the business.

Do-it-yourself sellers should go to Owners.com. This site, which has merged with Homebytes.com, offers over 25,000 "For Sale by Owner" (FSBO, pronounced "fizbo") home listings. In 2000, 1,000,000 U.S. homeowners sold their homes by themselves.

A new generation of Internet-based realtors is emerging as viable competition to the traditional realtors and their full-commission arrangements. Two of the largest are eRealty.com and zipRealty.com. For example, eRealty.com offers a 1% rebate off the purchase price when you buy a home through one of their home-based realtors. In addition, eRealty.com will sell your home for a 4.5% maximum commission, considerably less than most traditional realtors. One of the best features of the new Internet-based realtors is their willingness to give consumers access to MLS data. At this time, eRealty.com and zipRealty.com operate only in certain major metropolitan areas. Even with their current limited market penetration, the real estate trends created by these firms are likely to gain increased consumer attention. Even eBay.com, the large Internet auctioneer, has gotten into Internet-based real estate sales. Having purchased

HomesDirect.com, a company that focused on foreclosed real estate, eBay.com now auctions off foreclosed homes and other properties from its popular Web site.

Yet another option now available to home buyers and sellers on the Web is "fee-for-service," which gives the homeowner a choice of how much help he or she wants from the realtor. Typically, if you want your listing included in the local MLS system, you will pay more than if you don't. In addition, the more work the realtor does, the more you will pay. If this type of arrangement appeals to you, two Web sites to explore are blueedge.com and helpusell.com. Not all locations are currently served by these firms.

Internet Home Shopping: The Future

The real future of Internet-based home shopping may involve intelligent on-line search engines now under development. These search engines will allow consumers to perform comprehensive real estate searches and will automatically match buyers with sellers without the involvement of any realtors. This search system, based on something called XML (extensible markup language), is getting the attention of some deep-pocketed firms including eBay. Basically, XML is a much more advanced search tool than most Internet search engines. While still in its infancy, an XML-based on-line real estate market certainly creates visions of a marketplace in which real estate transactions occur light-years faster than in our current system. Instead of taking months for real estate transactions to play out, the process of buying or selling real estate soon may more closely resemble trading shares of stock on-line. Already, we are seeing realtors as well as consumers using wireless Internet-enabled hand-held devices to look up and locate real estate information and directions on-line when physically searching for the ideal home. The possibilities are endless!

Of course, virtually all traditional real estate brokers, not to be upstaged, now have Web sites. Although the Internet has done a tremendous amount to put real estate information such as MLS listings in the hands of consumers, most serious home buyers and sellers may still be best served by both the Internet and the services of a real estate professional. The successful real estate professional of the future will embrace the Internet and other forms of technology as important tools to better serve real estate buyers and sellers. The Internet will continue to shape the real estate business for many years to come, but probably the most exciting benefit by far will be that more and more people will be able to identify the home of their dreams in less time for the best price.

HOME OWNERSHIP WEB SITES:

- www.bestplaces.net
- www.digitalcity.com
- www.ebay.com
- www.homeadvisor.com
- www.homebid.com
- www.homegain.com
- www.homes.com
- www.homestore.com
- www.imove.com
- www.monstermoving.com
- www.owners.com
- www.Realtor.com

Step 7: Mortgage Shopping, New Economy Style

As with buying real estate, the Internet has changed the way people shop for mortgages. So, the first step in shopping for your mortgage should be in educating yourself about current mortgage rates, the most appropriate mortgage for your situation, and the mortgage-buying process. The best place to start with this process is the Internet. By using the Internet as an information resource for mortgages, you can do your research when it's most convenient for you—and you just may find the best mortgage for your circumstances on the Web. I strongly encourage you explore all of the resources of the Internet first, even if you've never been on-line before. Here are some basic mortgage-related terms and costs you should be familiar with:

CLOSING COSTS: AN AVALANCHE OF FEES

Closing costs are the costs associated with transferring ownership of the home to you. Closings may take place at a title company, a bank, or an attorney's or realtor's office. We are now seeing the emergence of on-line real estate closings, which will significantly alter the real estate closing process. These are common costs that may be included with closing on your home:

- Transfer and recording taxes
- Title insurance
- Site survey fee
- Appraisal fees
- Credit report fee
- Settlement or closing fees
- Termite inspection
- Application fee
- Processing fee
- Loan discount points
- Real estate broker commissions
- Attorney's fees
- Fees for preparing the legal documents

As you can see, there are many different types of fees that you can be charged when buying or selling a home. Some of the closing fees will be paid by the buyer and some will be paid by the seller. One very valuable lesson I learned about closing fees and closing agreements is to get them in writing before you attend the closing. Have the title company or closing attorney involved fax or e-mail you the documents at least one day before the formal closing so that you can read the closing documents (and learn about all the fees) at your leisure and make sure all your questions are answered before the closing takes place. If there is something you do not completely understand, ask until you do! In addition to getting your questions answered, you won't feel pressured at the closing. Closing costs are generally 2% to 6% of the sales price of your home, not including the real estate broker's commissions, which can run as high as 7% of the sales price.

Points

Points, also known as discount points, are a fee paid to the mortgage lender. One point equals 1% of the loan amount. For example, one point on a $100,000 loan is $1,000. Points represent extra money you can pay the lender at closing in exchange for a lower interest rate loan. Usually, the longer you plan to stay in your home, the more sense it makes to pay points. Points are generally considered to be tax-deductible.

NON-CONFORMING LOANS

Non-conforming loans are also known as jumbo loans. Generally, if you are borrowing over $322,700, the current limit set for conforming loans by the Federal National Mortgage Association (FNMA) and the Federal Home Loan Mortgage Corporation (FHLMC), you may be required to make a larger down payment and you may also pay a higher interest rate.

PRIVATE MORTGAGE INSURANCE

Private Mortgage Insurance (PMI) is a financial guarantee that protects mortgage lenders against loss if the borrower defaults. In order to avoid paying private mortgage insurance you will be required to make at least a 20% down payment. Once the equity in your home reaches 20%, you will no longer have to pay PMI. However, it is solely your responsibility to notify the lender when this figure has been reached.

Instead of making a 20% down payment, there are a couple of creative ways to avoid paying PMI, which typically costs $25–$150 per month for a median-priced home. One strategy is to obtain a first mortgage for 80% of the value of your home and have the lender also provide a 15% home-equity second mortgage. You would then make a 5% cash down payment at closing. This is called an 80–15–5. You can also do something similar using an 80–10–10, where a 10% home equity second mortgage and 10% cash down payment are used with an 80% first mortgage. An alternative in both cases to obtaining a second mortgage from a lender is to have the seller carry the second mortgage.

—*Mortgages and the Internet*—

In the year 2000 about one trillion dollars worth of mortgage loans were made. Only $20 billion of these loans were closed with on-line Internet providers. Does this mean that on-line mortgage companies are doomed? Definitely not! Gomez Advisors, an Internet research firm in Lincoln, Massachusetts, says that about 50% of all home-buyers now go on-line as a first step to home-buying information, such as mortgages. That's up from 12% two years ago, and this growth trend is expected to continue.

As mortgage information provided on-line becomes more accessible with better content, the public will increasingly take advantage of this fast and inexpensive way to research interest rates and other pertinent mortgage information.

The Mortgage Application Process

The mortgage loan application process will require you to provide some information, for example:

- Borrower's and co-borrower's personal information (address, phone numbers, social security numbers, etc.)

- Your adjusted gross income from all sources, as well as your job stability

- Your current debt, including auto loans, credit cards, personal loans, household expenses, etc.

Before you make your formal mortgage loan application, I suggest checking with the three major credit agencies to see for yourself what your credit reports look like. It is quite common to find mistakes on your credit reports or issues that should be resolved before making your mortgage application. Here are the three major credit reporting agencies:

- Equifax.com 1-800-685-1111

- Experian.com 1-888-397-3742

- Transunion.com 1-800-888-4213

If you want to see how the major credit reporting agencies have evaluated your credit, go to www.myfico.com (there is a cost for this service).

While a vast storehouse of mortgage information is available on-line, the mortgage loan application process is not something everyone wants to do—or should do—via the Internet without professional guidance. For many mortgage buyers, the best approach is to utilize both on-line and human resources to come up with the best mortgage solution to meet their needs. Yes, do your research thoroughly on-line, getting as much information as you can before selecting your mortgage lender of choice. If you are an experienced mortgage shopper or want to shop for your mortgage via the Internet, completing the process on-line could save you some real cash by eliminating some of the costly fees listed in the closing costs section. In addition, Internet-based lender's rates are often below non-Internet lender's rates, sometimes by as much as a quarter percentage point. However, if you don't feel completely comfortable doing it yourself, get a mortgage professional involved to guide you through the process. Many of the on-line mortgage lenders are now offering the advice of a mortgage professional at no additional charge. You may not get the same feeling as if your mortgage advisor were sitting down the block from you; but then again; it may not matter, as long as you can save some money on fees and get a better rate. Make your choice based on what best meets your needs and what combination of services appeals to you the most. Here are some useful mortgage information Web sites:

USEFUL MORTGAGE WEB SITES

- www.E-Loan.com
- www.Mortgage.com
- www.Indymac.com

- www.Lendingtree.com
- www.Countrywide.com
- www.Loansdirect.com

—*The Future of Real Estate*—

The Internet has dramatically and permanently changed the home-buying experience. Those who have not yet realized the powerful force of the Internet on the real estate business will inevitably do so in the future. The changes the real estate industry faces as a result of increased use of technology are long-term trends that are accelerating at a rapid pace.

The enormous amount of real estate information provided by the Internet will result in a more highly educated consumer and, we can hope, a more consumer-oriented real estate professional, who will be required to provide more valuable and more diverse services to the real estate client. The greatest benefit of the Internet's impact on the real estate business is that consumers will be able to buy and sell properties at the optimum price in the least amount of time.

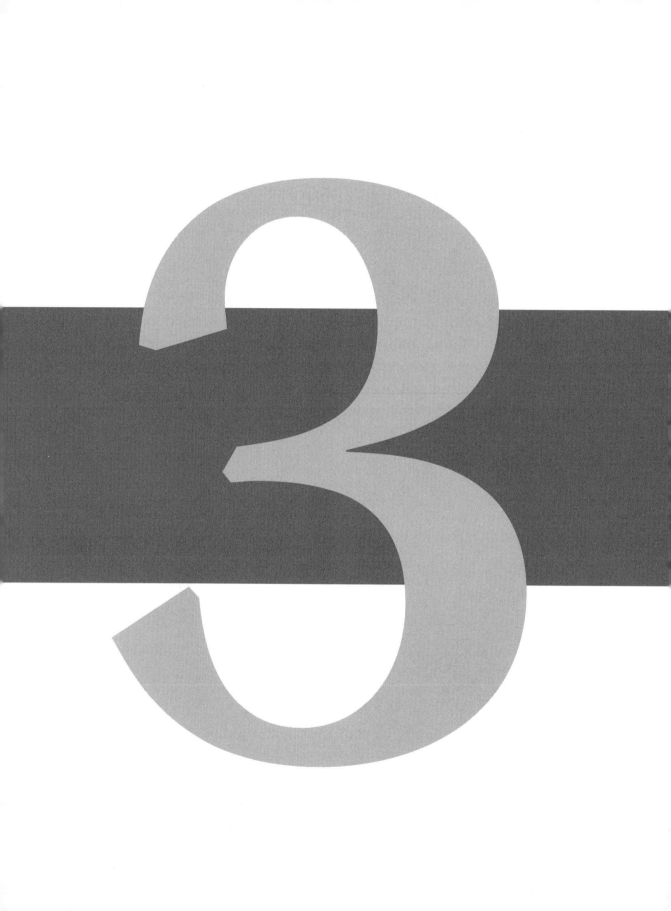

CHAPTER THREE

The Home-Based Business Revolution

The Home-Based Business Revolution

> *Do what you love and success will surely follow!*

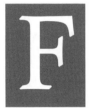or many years a radical change has been underway in the world of business. The hierarchical and bureaucratic organizational models left over from the Industrial Age have become obsolete relics, even though some companies, unwilling to change, have not completely accepted this fact as truth. Corporations that hold onto this outdated model will have trouble competing with the new "technology-based" organizational structure designed for rapid response to changing consumer demand.

Information technology, particularly Internet-related technologies, are still in their infancy in terms of their effect on how the world does business. Information technology has caused major productivity gains in most large corporations, particularly those that have moved away from a hierarchical business structure and embraced the new consumer-oriented "network" model. This new model focuses on utilizing technology in all phases of business, in order to better serve the fast-changing needs of consumers. Unfortunately, these giant leaps in productivity mean that, in many cases, fewer employees are required because technology has made each employee substantially more productive, eliminating the need for certain types of employees. In addition, the new Internet-based organization is substantially more efficient in its operation, requiring fewer employees to produce the same amount of goods or services than in an industrial-age-style corporation.

The economic downturn of the early 2000s merely accelerated the trend towards corporate hiring of fewer, more technologically savvy employees in an effort to further trim costs. In an economic downturn most companies are unable to increase sales, so the only recourse they have to improve profits is to cut costs, often by reducing the workforce. We must always remember one indisputable fact about corporations: their ultimate goal is to satisfy their stockholders, the owners of the corporation. Unfortunately, when forced to choose between the stockholders and the employees, corporations will first seek to gratify the shareholders' desire for greater profits, which many times results in lost jobs.

As evidence of the trend towards rapid job cutting by corporations eager to reduce costs, outplacement firm Challenger, Gray & Christmas reported that in December of 2001, 22,000 jobs were eliminated in the U.S. in a little over 24 hours. Not only is this an incredibly large number in a short period of time, but it also confirms a disturbing precedent that firing workers between the Thanksgiving and New Year Holiday season is no longer taboo but perfectly acceptable. This is further solid evidence of rapidly declining employer-employee trust and relationships.

In this new, technologically advanced business environment, major corporations are banking on the premise that the new "techno-employee" will embrace these changes and view them as ultimately positive. Furthermore, they believe that these employees will then recognize the changes as a means of increasing the company's competitive position, thereby creating an enriched work environment. The reality is that the employees who remain are being asked to carry a greater workload to compensate for a smaller number of employees overall. This in turn causes increased stress and a less desirable lifestyle for many employees.

Big corporations spend a great deal of time and money convincing employees of their personal importance to the corporation. Many proclaim, "Our employees are our most important resource." Of course, conventional wisdom says that if you please both consumers and employees, sales (and, hopefully, profits) will naturally rise, thus satisfying stockholders. Many CEOs (yes, there are many honorable CEOs) would like to please everyone. However, the breathtaking speed of changes in the marketplace, a result of instantaneous global access to information, has forced changes that many CEOs understandably have a difficult time coping with; and some CEOs (and their accountants) have resorted to fraudulent accounting methods as a way to increase profits.

—*Economic Megatrends*—

"I think the Internet is like electricity."
Michael S. Dell, CEO, Dell Computer Corporation

In many corporations, a distinct shift is currently underway, placing greater emphasis on pleasing consumers who want highly customized products and services at lower prices. Great pressure is put on corporations to satisfy these increasingly demanding consumers and to make a profit at the same time.

Direct-to-Consumer Business Model

It has been apparent for quite some time that the assembly line business model first popularized by Henry Ford in the early 1900s is obsolete and that the direct-to-consumer business model long advocated by Dell Computer is the successful business model of today. The direct business model does away with the middleman and delivers a fully customized product directly to the consumer. There is no retail store or inventory of products. In addition, the model lends itself to greater use of Internet shopping by consumers. You go online and customize your system exactly as you want it. All of these factors contribute to less employee overhead expense. Computer manufacturers that mass-produce computers Henry Ford-style are rapidly losing market share to Dell. Because Dell operates with a much lower cost structure than the competition, it can squeeze competitors and win any price war it wants to engage in. Dell has established the competitive terms of engagement and can therefore pick and choose the types of market share it most wants to gain.

Another industry that is quickly realizing the superiority of the direct-to-consumer business model is none other than the automobile industry. The auto industry is currently going through some of the most massive changes since the automobile was invented. The government is pushing what it calls the "freedom car," a vehicle designed to reduce reliance on foreign oil (particularly Middle Eastern oil) by encouraging the auto industry to develop hydrogen-powered cars. Regardless of the types of cars the auto makers ultimately manufacture, the old system of mass-producing automobiles and sending them off to a dealer's lot where they sit until a salesman can persuade someone to buy one of them is quickly becoming obsolete.

The Dell model of customized, direct-to-consumer manufacturing will undoubtedly gain popularity in the automotive world, too. You can now purchase autos online through various sites such as Autobytel.com and CarsDirect.com. Of course, most people will want to test drive the cars they are buying, but the number of auto dealerships in existence today seems excessive.

Because of the vast amount of information available instantaneously, the Internet exposes inefficiencies in business models and will force companies and industries to adapt to the most efficient way. The new economic megatrend of greater numbers of consumers buying online rather than through retail establishments also has implications for the commercial real estate market. If large numbers of consumers do begin to buy substantially more products online, this may happen at the expense not only of retail merchants in strip centers and shopping malls but also auto dealerships. In turn, this retail business downturn could adversely affect the price of commercial real estate. While issues like this do involve local real estate conditions, and each real estate market does have unique characteristics, the commercial real estate market as a whole could suffer.

The lack of high-quality workers in the late 1990s, resulting in one of the best environments employees have ever seen, caused a backlash in which big corporations accelerated the use of technology in an effort to reduce employee overhead. Employment is the single biggest expense for many companies, particularly service-oriented businesses. A major sector of technology that is currently booming is computer-based customer relationship management (CRM) software. This software is designed to reduce human intervention in the customer service process, with a side benefit of reducing employee overhead for corporations. The notion that computers serve only to increase worker productivity, not to eliminate some of them, is purely a myth. Permanently diminishing the workforce has now become a major goal of many large corporations.

—U.S. Employees Replaced by Global Workforce—

There is another threat U.S. employees must concern themselves with in the Digital Age. While traditional corporate downsizings and technological innovation are part of today's business environment, a major global trend has been developing that could eventually deliver a further blow to the job security of many Americans: the non-traditional, methodical process of firing U.S. workers and replacing them with employees in places like China (population 1.3 billion, according to the China Population Information and Research Center), India (over 1 billion people), eastern Europe, South Africa, and many other developing areas around the globe. U.S. corporations are attracted to foreign workers who are college-educated—many with doctorates—schooled in fields like engineering, architecture, accounting, technology, financial services, and biotechnology. For example, the Philippines turns out 380,000 college graduates per year; India already has over 500,000 information technology engineers, and the starting annual salary for an Indian engineer is $5,000. In the financial services industry U.S. firms are expected to replace 500,000 U.S. workers, or 8% of industry employment, with foreign workers by 2008, with a prospective savings of $30 billion (source: management consultant A. T. Kearney).

While some U.S. workers face the elimination of their jobs, others will experience a less familiar and possibly longer-lasting problem: decreased pay and reduced benefits. The circumstances behind the arrival of the new "no-raise employee" are similar to those of the jobless; technological innovation, weak economic conditions, deflationary pressures, and a formidable—and less expensive—global workforce. The typical job search for an unemployed American is now five months, a 19-year high. According to the outplacement firm Challenger, Gray, & Christmas, the 17% of the workforce that do find work are accepting reduced pay (twice the historical norm). In addition, 80% of employers intend to place more of the burden for health insurance costs on the remaining employees (Kaiser Family Foundation, 2003).

Since the boom times of the late 1990s, a fundamental shift in employer attitudes regarding employees has occurred. Employees are increasingly seen as short-term commodities to be used or discarded as business conditions dictate. The stark reality of U.S. employment in the 21st century is that technology has advanced to the point where one employee can now do the job that previously required the services of many; and, as we have seen, the work can be performed anywhere in the world.

Even though good-paying jobs, especially for the technologically savvy, will continue to exist, the pressures and stresses of these jobs will be enormous. The goals of lowering the costs of employee overhead through increased use of technology and communications and of hiring more global workers have risen to the forefront of the war to win shareholder satisfaction in the 21st century. The major casualty of this war will continue to be the employee. However, the obvious question is—what will become of many of these displaced employees? The answer is that many will never return to the traditional workplace. Instead, a new breed of 21st-century entrepreneurs is rapidly emerging.

—A New Entrepreneur Emerges—

"I think there is a world market for maybe five computers."
Thomas Watson, IBM Chairman, 1943

Throughout the history of business, there has always been a correlation between prosperity and information access. During the early 1980s, the personal computer became widely available and affordable, which resulted in the ability of much of the population to process information at a greater speed. The personal computer began a major trend towards enabling large numbers of people to do things that previously only large corporations could accomplish using multi-million-dollar mainframe computers. Another major trend that began to blossom at that time was the development of home-based businesses.

Advancements in communications and Internet technologies since the late 1990s have been incredible. Today, the instantaneous access to information and our ability to communicate that information are light years from where it was just a few short years ago. E-mail, cellular phones, broadband communications, high-speed Internet access, satellite transmission, vast networks of computers, and instant messaging have put the power of information in the hands of the people. This technological revolution has bred a new class of entrepreneur, armed with low-cost Internet and cellular technologies and reaping the tremendous benefits of operating from a home office. This is a trend that is still in its infancy, but it will surely revolutionize the way the world does business.

The Time of Your Life

"Dost thou love life? Then do not squander time,
for that is the stuff life is made of."
Benjamin Franklin

According to a 2003 study by Texas A&M University's Texas Transportation Institute that examined traffic congestion in 68 urban areas, in 2001 the average American spent 51 hours stuck in traffic. That means stuck *motionless* in traffic. That's more than three times the levels seen in 1982. I'm sure that inhaling exhaust fumes while sitting in stalled traffic during the commute to your job isn't the most pleasant experience you could imagine at 7:00 A.M. The Texas A&M traffic study does not take into account time spent actually driving to the job (when the traffic is moving) in their traffic congestion figures. To illustrate just how much time is being wasted, let's look at an example. If, including time stuck in traffic, your one-way commute to your office or workplace is 30 minutes, your round-trip time totals one hour. In a five-day workweek that's five hours a week. Multiply that by 50 weeks and you have an astounding 250 hours wasted in commuting to and from work each year—the equivalent of over six full weeks of work wasted driving to and from work, time most employers will not pay you for. Neither does your employer pay you for gas and oil, repairs, tolls, and all the costs involved in owning or leasing your automobile. In addition, many employers today require some weekend work, and most employees still get only between two and four weeks of vacation annually.

The bottom line is that employees have little financial security and face an enormous amount of work-related stress and job dissatisfaction. If all of this weren't enough, you can be fired from your job at any time if you don't have an employment contract.

There really is no gold watch worth waiting for after many years of sacrifice at a job. Your time is very valuable because you are a very valuable person with unique skills and talents. Think of all the things you could do with six extra weeks a year. Time is the one thing we absolutely cannot get back once it is gone.

The True Meaning of Success

Today, what people want most is a balanced lifestyle in which a successful career is just one component of a happy, successful, and rewarding life. While having financial resources is certainly important, being successful is much more than material wealth. It's about having true friends who can pour their hearts out to you when they're feeling down. It's about creating exciting win-win solutions for everyone (win-lose is just so terribly wrong). It's about being healthy in mind, body, and spirit and associating with positive and uplifting people. It's about feeling good about who you are and where you are going in life. It's about believing in unlimited possibilities and creating a fabulous lifestyle with someone you love.

We want the best of all worlds—and after all, why shouldn't we have it? People want the opportunity to see their kids grow up and to watch them play baseball or participate in their ballet lessons. We want the freedom to pursue the occupation that best fits our personalities and goals. We'd like more leisure time to spend on hobbies we enjoy or travel to places we'd always dreamed of. We want to live in a location and home that best suits our lifestyle. We want the opportunity to make interesting new friends and spend more time with our families. In essence, what we really want is greater control over our lives, which means having the necessary finances, having total confidence in yourself and having the available time to do what you please.

—Home-Based Businesses Expand Rapidly—

All kinds of people from all different types of backgrounds are joining the home-based business revolution:

- Baby-boomers and Generation Xers who are sick and tired of having a boss and want more out of life than a dead-end career

- Generation Y "20-somethings" who, unlike their baby-boomer parents, learned how to use computers in nursery school and choose to use the power of the information to their greatest avantage

- A growing number of enterprising college and graduate students planning to bypass the corporate route altogether

- Retired people armed with empowering technology and rejuvenated spirits who want to begin a new business, possibly started from an existing hobby

- Single mothers and housewives who want to stay home for their children and still have rewarding careers

- Professionals such as doctors (MDs, chiropractors, psychologists, acupuncturists, and other natural health-care physicians), lawyers, accountants, financial advisors, realtors, and dentists who realize that the increased legal regulations, malpractice insurance costs, mountains of paperwork, and expensive employee overhead require putting in longer and longer hours just to make the same amount of income

- High-level executives who are tired of the corporate politics, constant traveling, overwhelming job responsibilities, unhealthy stress, and lack of time to do much else

- Small-business owners who are tired of paying for outrageously overpriced office space and want to reduce overhead expenses in general to create a more balanced lifestyle and have the time to enjoy it

- Workers in high-rise office buildings (and all other office buildings) and those who commute by airplane and have concerns for their safety and the welfare of their families

Home-based businesses in one form or another are becoming the solution for many U.S. workers in the 21st century. The trend continues to develop because of loss of jobs and pay cuts. In addition, due to surging demand many new homes today come with a "home office" as a standard feature.

According to International Data Corporation, the average income for home-based business households is $59,000 annually, compared to an average annual income of about $42,000 for all Americans (U.S. Census Bureau). Therefore, home-based business owners earn about 29% more income than the average American household.

Startup capital, expenses, legal regulations, and government-required paperwork for traditional businesses have made the costs of establishing a traditional business prohibitive for most Americans. Franchises can easily cost $250,000 or more just for the right to use a name, and that doesn't even include the cost of buying or renting real estate, paying employees (including benefits), and other expensive items of overhead required by these types of businesses.

Home-Based Business Owner Satisfaction

Consider some interesting statistics regarding home-based business owners in the USA:

- 86% of all home-based business owners are happier owning their own businesses than being an employee

- 125,000 Americans start a home-based business every week

- 20% reported gross sales between $100,000 and $500,000 (less than 5% of all employees earn over $100,000 annually)

- 29% of home-based business owners work with family members

- 33% of all new millionaires own a home-based business

—*Employee Tax Burden*—

According to a 2003 study by the Washington, D.C.-based Tax Foundation, American taxpayers in the year 2003 had to work from January 1st until April 19th—the 109th day of the year—before earning enough money to meet their annual tax obligations. According to Scott Hodge, executive director of the Tax Foundation, "Americans will work longer to pay for government in 2003 than they will for food, clothing, and shelter combined."

If you are an employee in the United States today, your employment gives you little in the way of tax advantages. Your income is fully taxable with minimal if any business tax deductions.

—*Home-Based Business Advantages*—

There are numerous advantages to owning your own home-based business. Here are just a few of the reasons so many people are developing this lifestyle:

- Typically, start-up costs are very low.

- Smart use of technology minimizes the need for expensive employees.

- You will have no state or federal employee-related paperwork.

- Not commuting to an office saves time and gas and lowers auto expenses.

- Not commuting gives you more time to sleep and thus improves your health.

- Not having to commute by air saves tremendous amounts of time and money, particularly in these days of travel delays due to increased airline security measures.

- Home offices require no expensive office leases or additional utility expenses.

- Having your office in your home eliminates concerns about an office away from home.

- You can be there to raise your family plus have your own career.

- You control your time and the hours you work.

- You have the freedom to determine how much income you want to earn.

- No office politics.

- You are under less stress from employers who are trying to squeeze more work out of fewer employees.

- Computers, fax machines, and all equipment are under your control.

- You can carve out more time for family and friends.

- You can create the business that best fits into your ultimate lifestyle.

- You can benefit from tremendous tax advantages (see page 79).

Moving the Office into the Home

*Ditch the traditional office and
move up to a bigger and better home.*

If you have usually worked from an office outside your home or have family or other dependents living at home, you may be wondering if a home-based business would work for you. One factor to consider in your decision is how much more home you can afford if you eliminate the expense of an outside office. For example, let's say that an office outside your home would cost you $600 per month, a very conservative amount today. Also, let's assume that your office commute is 30 minutes each way for a total of a one-hour commute, and your monthly gasoline bill is $65. This too is a conservative estimate, especially since we are not adding in the cost of tolls, insurance, and the maintenance of your automobile. That's a total of $665 per month you would save ($600 + $65 = $665).

If your current home is too small to accommodate your new home office, consider adding an office wing on to your existing home or buying a new home altogether. With that extra $665 per month, you can now afford a much larger and nicer home—about $100,000 nicer. Yes, a $100,000 30-year fixed-rate mortgage at 7% will cost you about $665 per month. In addition, nothing says that you have to use the entire mortgage on office space. How about using some of that mortgage money on a bigger, more modern kitchen with granite countertops, a new deck with a pool, or a home gym? The good news doesn't stop there; you should also factor in the many substantial tax advantages you will enjoy from having your office in your home. If you are like me and a growing number of Americans, you already have some type of office in your home. So why duplicate expenses such as phone lines, office equipment, and furniture when you can centralize all of your operations in the comfort of your own home? When you add up all of the advantages—such as transportation savings (gas, auto, tolls, repair, etc.), time savings, tax advantages, and the chance to move up to a bigger and better home—there isn't much of a question, financial or otherwise, as to which is the better choice. And after all, wouldn't you prefer to get all the tax write-offs and pay off your own mortgage instead of paying off the landlord's mortgage?

Flexible, Low-Cost Office Space: Designed for Today's Technologies

It stands to reason that there may come a time when you need occasional office space to meet with clients or for some other business purpose. This is still no reason to pay your landlord's mortgage for overpriced office space. Today a growing number of office building owners are eager to rent out conference rooms or excess office space by the hour or the day. I have seen office space in upscale office buildings that can be rented for $15 an hour. It has increasingly become a buyer's market for office space since the Internet bubble burst. Concerns about the safety of office buildings have also worked to the benefit of consumers.

Many of today's newly outfitted office buildings have technology-ready offices and conference rooms where you can bring your portable computer, plug it in to a high-speed Internet port, and you're ready to work. Also, many office buildings are installing inexpensive and easy-to-use Wi-Fi (wireless fidelity) technology access points that allow computer users the freedom of wireless connection to the Internet.

With better technologies and falling prices for cellular phones and wireless Internet access, fixed-line phones and cabled computers are becoming obsolete in the new business model of the Digital Age. Businesses are quickly moving toward greater cell phone and wireless Internet usage to eliminate the extra cost, duplication, inflexibility, and immobility associated with fixed-line phones, and cabled computers.

Attempt to do as much of your business as you can from your home office. It will save you a tremendous amount of time and money. However, if you need additional space, a growing amount of inexpensive, "flexible" office space is available to suit your needs.

—The Wireless Mobile Information Society—

The changes taking place today in technology, business, and society are staggering. Nowhere is this more evident than in the movement towards small, lightweight, portable, wireless electronic devices that allow business people in America and around the globe to literally carry their offices with them. People can now utilize a "mobile office" or "virtual office" approach to their careers. At the forefront of this technology in the new mobilized information society is something called a "communicator," a device about the size of a cellular phone that allows for a variety of capabilities in one unit. At your fingertips is a cellular phone, a personal digital assistant, and a good-sized screen that allows you to surf the Web plus send and receive e-mails all in one device. Many communicators now have in-built keyboards so that the user can quickly write memos or e-mails, and some even include PC functionality. In addition, you can synchronize data such as client contact information between your PC and your communicator by plugging the communicator into the USB port on the back of your computer. Many communicators now allow you to synchronize your data through a wireless Internet connection. Some devices have voice recognition, allowing you to dial phone numbers or call up important client data on the screen simply with the sound of your voice.

In addition to desiring all-in-one business functionality on wireless handheld devices, consumers apparently want to be entertained as well. In a recent HPI Research Group Study, 72% of respondents said that they would prefer to have at least one mobile entertainment service on their wireless handheld device. Radio, live TV, digital photography, on-demand music, and video games were some of the most popular entertainment features.

Another exciting benefit of the new wireless devices is facilitation of Global Positioning System (GPS) technology, which uses satellite communications to provide information such as maps of the user's current location and the most efficient travel route to the user's destination. Voice technology can give you the directions verbally. The new GPS systems can also map trails for travel guides, hikers, and backpackers and can even locate fish for both commercial and recreational purposes.

In essence, the new wireless communications devices promise to completely transform the way we do business and where we do it. The days of being chained to a desk for eight to ten hours a day because of technological restrictions are over. For those starting a new home-based business, the types of technological innovations I am describing will allow for greater freedom of movement and a tremendous time savings that will allow you to be in touch with your clients (and anyone else) at any time you choose at any location on the planet. Just think of the possibilities!

—*Home-Based Business Tax Advantages*—

One of the most significant advantages to a home-based business is the vast array of tax deductions you can claim. Here are just some of the business expenses you may deduct from your taxable income as a home-based business owner:

- Business start-up costs (costs incurred before business began; research, travel, consultant fee, etc.)
- Advertising
- Auto expenses
- Educational expenses
- Meals and entertainment
- Computers, cell phones, fax machines, printers, and all other office equipment
- Office furniture and supplies

- Publications
- Repairs and maintenance
- Taxes and licenses
- Travel
- Bank fees on business accounts
- Business gifts

Home Office Deductions

The "home office deduction" is one of the best tax advantages for your home-based business. This deduction is actually a number of deductions that are reported on IRS Form 8829, "Expenses for Business Use of Your Home." Here are some common home office deductions:

- Mortgage payments for the portion of the home used for a home office

- The percentage of homeowner's insurance used for the home office

- Heat, air conditioning and electrical expenses used for the home office

- Trash collection, security systems services and cleaning services as a percentage of your home office usage

- Business telephone charges including home phone and cellular phone (A second phone line used strictly for business may be deducted 100%.)

- Home office repairs and decorating expenses

- Home office burglary or casualty losses (hurricane, flood, fire, accident or vandalism)

If you rent your home, you may also deduct the portion of your rental payments that pertain to your home office.

In order to qualify for the home office deductions, your home office *must be used exclusively and regularly for business* and either 1) be your "principal place of business" or be normally used to personally meet with clients *or* 2) be a separate structure that is not attached to your house or residence, in which case it merely has to be used in your trade or business.

Need Some Help? Hire the Kids

One frequently overlooked tax break for home-based business owners is hiring your children under age 18 and deducting their salary as a business expense. There are three tests the IRS uses to determine the eligibility of the "kiddie deduction":

- First, all payments must be of a reasonable amount. To determine what's reasonable, figure out what you would normally pay a non-related employee to perform the same task.

- Second, your child must do business-related tasks. If the IRS deems the work to be household chores or other non-business related work you will not get the deduction.

- Third, your child must be an employee on the payroll. You will be responsible for reporting Social Security, unemployment, and Medicare taxes.

Be sure to keep employment records as you would for any other employees. In fact, keeping additional records that list all of the tasks performed is a good idea here.

There's actually a second tax break associated with the kiddie deduction: $3,000 of the child's pay may go into a tax-free Roth IRA to begin the child's "nest egg." This is a good way of teaching your children the value of investing for the future. It is sure to give them a great sense of accomplishment and give you, the parent, some welcome help with your business and taxes.

—*Types of Home-Based Businesses*—

Essentially, home-based businesses, whether Internet-based or not, fall into three categories: fee-for-service, product sales, and network marketing.

Fee-for-Service

In a fee-for-service home-based business, you charge either an hourly rate or a flat fee for services you perform. Basically, with fee-for-service you get paid for the time worked whether the client is paying an hourly fee or a flat rate for the complete job. Examples of fee-for-service home-based businesses are graphic design, Internet web site design, legal services, health-care insurance forms preparation, and accounting services.

Fee-for-service home-based businesses are inherently limiting. This is because your income is limited to the time you have available, and you have only 24 hours in a day (and I'm sure you don't want to be working for most of them). Therefore, there is little opportunity to leverage your time.

Traditional Product Sales

In home-based businesses involved in product sales, products are bought at whole-sale and sold at retail. Of course, the difference between the wholesale and retail prices is the gross profit on the sale. The increased use of the Internet has resulted in many more people selling in this manner; however with greater competition comes increased pricing pressure on retail sales prices. So, while it is generally easier to sell more products through the Internet, actually making enough of a profit to make it all worthwhile is another story altogether. Probably the most popular example of the difficulty of generating profits through on-line retail sales is Amazon.com, the largest on-line retailer in the world, which never had a problem selling products like books, electronics, and toys, but found that actually making a profit was a much more difficult task. However, in recent times Amazon.com, along with major Internet players eBay and Yahoo!, have experienced explosive growth and improved profitability. All of these companies exemplify the rewards of perseverance and the ever-increasing power of the Internet.

As with fee-for-service home-based businesses, home-based businesses based on product sales have limitations—in this case, a "linear" type of arrangement where one product sold generates one profit with no additional benefits. Another major issue facing these businesses is that increased price competition from other companies using the Internet makes it tough to make a profit.

The Internet has the ability in itself to make many products into "commodities," which, in turn, lowers prices. It is a fabulous tool for lowering inflation but requires ever more innovative and skillful marketing for product sales entrepreneurs to make a profit.

Network Marketing

"I would rather have 1% of the efforts of 100 people than 100% of my own efforts."
J. Paul Getty

Network marketing, otherwise known as "multi-level marketing," is a form of product distribution in which the marketing of all products and services is performed by the consumers of the products and services instead of by the "company."

The foundation of network marketing is built upon the people who form the network. The network grows as more and more consumers of the product or service share their experience with others, primarily through word-of-mouth advertising. The network grows in a geometric fashion. Consumers in the network promote the opportunity to others, which, in turn, builds the organization ("downline") larger and larger. Probably the best example of how network marketing works is to think of how you would tell someone about a good movie you saw or a great restaurant with wonderful food and atmosphere, or even a good book you just read. For instance, let's say that you tell three other people about your fabulous products and they join the network. In turn, those three people tell three other people, and so on. The major attraction of network marketing for the home-based business entrepreneur is the potential for unlimited growth of the network, which could mean an unlimited income for you.

Linear vs. Residual Income

Traditional home-based businesses work on the premise of linear income—working for a fixed hourly fee or through finite product sales. Even though many traditional business owners make very good incomes, the income is limited to how many hours they can work. It's essentially a time-for-money trap. If you are in home-based product sales, your income is also limited, because, although you may be able to generate lots of sales, the only way to increase sales dramatically is by increasing overhead (employees, inventory, equipment, etc.), which is exactly what most home-based business owners were trying to escape to begin with.

Network marketing approaches the subject of income in a dramatically different way. The major difference comes from how the income is derived. Rather than relying solely on your own efforts to increase your income, with network marketing your efforts are multiplied by the efforts of the other people in your organization. You derive compensation from the sales made by all of the people in your network. You are therefore "leveraging" your efforts by teaching others how to do what you are doing. In essence, it's a win-win proposition, utilizing the principle of duplication. Therefore, with network marketing you may generate a never-ending stream of residual income, income that comes in month after month, year after year, as long as the network remains healthy and strong.

As with other home-based businesses, network marketing allows you to do away with the daily round-trip commute, enjoy a more flexible schedule, reduce overhead costs, and allow more time with family and friends. However, network marketing offers benefits far beyond those of most home-based businesses:

- Very low start-up costs

- Little or no business risk

- Opportunity to truly help people while helping yourself

- A business which you can pass on to your children

- Greater personal growth for yourself

- Creation of win-win relationships

- Making friends for life

- A return to old-fashioned business values

- The great feeling you have about your career and yourself

- Opportunity for unlimited income

Choosing a Network Marketing Company

Once you have made the decision to become involved in a home-based network marketing venture, make sure you investigate the company thoroughly. Here's what I recommend you look for:

- **Top-quality consumable products.** Make sure that the offerings from the company are of top quality and will stand the test of time. As a general rule, look for companies with products that people will use over and over again, such as personal care or home care products or nutritional supplements.

- **Good management.** The top executives of the company should share your values regarding ethical management and commitment to excellence.

- **Expert opinion.** What are the industry experts saying about the company? During your research, learn to separate fact from fiction.

- **Track record.** How long has the company been in business? Have there been any complaints of a consistent or recurring nature from consumers in the network? Every growing company will experience some legal problems and complaints in this litigious society, so be sure to keep this in perspective.

- **Reach out and touch someone.** Call up the company's main headquarters and ask to speak with several of the company's executives. Evaluate them on their own merit.

- **Prominent affiliations.** Does the company retain on staff any experts prominent in their particular industry who can add credibility and invaluable expertise? This can often be a major coup for many fast-growing companies, sometimes making the difference between success and failure.

- **Compensation system.** Have a member of the network or someone from the home office's support staff fully explain the payment plan to you. After all, no matter how personally rewarding your experience will be, you're going to want to be paid for your efforts.

In the final analysis, after examining one or more network marketing companies, you are going to eventually have to make a gut-level decision. Above all else, make certain you *feel good* about your choice. Remember, this is *your* choice. You will be the one doing the work and reaping the rewards.

—*The Reality of Selling*—

Selling is simply believing in something so deeply and passionately that you have an overwhelming desire to tell others about it.

Anyone who aspires to be an entrepreneur will ultimately have to sell something. Whether you realize it or not, you are "selling yourself" every day of your life. Unfortunately, the words "sales," "sell," or "selling" have taken on a negative connotation in American society. The word "sell" conjures up visions of a pushy and irritating sales person who won't take "no" for answer. Therefore, many people who might otherwise have become great entrepreneurs did not because they thought they couldn't sell or they didn't want to be pushy. Selling and being pushy have absolutely nothing in common.

Unfortunately, many people around the world have a distorted understanding of what selling really is. The *American Heritage Dictionary* defines the word "sell" as "to persuade another to recognize worth or desirability." Yes, it's true. However, some sales people are persuasive to the point of being offensive. In any event, the dictionary's definition of selling falls far short of the real definition.

To truly understand what selling is, think of how a child persuades Mom or Dad to purchase ice cream or candy; or consider how anyone who really has a deep conviction or desire for you to understand and accept his or her way of thinking attempts to persuade you. Selling is simply believing in something so deeply and passionately that you have an overwhelming desire to tell others about it. Telling someone about a great movie you just saw is a good example. No one is paying you a dime to do it, but you are turning in a superb sales performance without even knowing it. Most people can tell instinctively whether you really believe in something or whether your motives are purely financial in nature.

Think about some of the great sales people of all time: people like Martin Luther King, Jr., and Sir Winston Churchill were great salespeople. Whether you agreed with them or liked them was irrelevant; what's important is that they were very persuasive and passionate about their causes.

The real problem most people experience with sales is that they don't truly believe in or have a passion for what they are promoting or selling. This actually results in a lose-lose situation. Salespersons attempting to persuade someone to purchase something they themselves do not believe in will not do a very good job at it, and the consumers will end up feeling as if they have encountered either a pushy or incompetent salesperson—a lose-lose proposition, all the way.

Most of us at one time or another have had the experience of working with those rare individuals who truly and passionately believed in what they were promoting. After the purchase, you felt as if you just had an extremely satisfying experience with a knowledgeable advisor who helped you make an important decision that was in your best interest. Isn't that an unusual occurrence these days? It doesn't have to be. You have the power within you to be a passionate and caring salesperson and to set a great example for everyone else!

Selling is nothing more than communicating your feelings about a product or service to other human beings. The entire difference is your true, deep-down feelings about what you are promoting and how you communicate that to others.

Go out and find a product or service you truly have a passion for and learn how to communicate the benefits effectively. Better yet, ask yourself what you like to do and think of how many other people might like to experience the same thing! You will be creating a win-win relationship with everyone you come in contact with, regardless of whether you experience an immediate financial benefit. The positive energy you create will ultimately result in greater benefits than you can imagine at this time.

—How to Start a Home-Based Business—

The idea of starting your own home-based business may seem like a daunting task, especially if you have been an employee for a long time and have never been self-employed. If you will just step out of your comfort zone and have confidence in your abilities, I'll help you do the rest. Here are the steps to take when starting your home-based business:

Step 1: Determine Your Product or Service

The first question you will have to answer when starting your home-based business is, "What valuable product or service will I provide?" If you haven't already decided this, just think about what you like to do, what you are passionate about. Why not do something that you enjoy, instead of forcing yourself to do something because you think you can make tons of money at it. There is real magic in doing what you love; others will sense it immediately. Many stressed-out executives and professionals who entered into careers because of the money wish they hadn't. Now some of those same people have decided to start their own home-based businesses. One other note of caution: be extremely careful if you are buying an existing business. If there are outstanding expenses or taxes owed to the IRS that you are unaware of, guess who just might end up paying those expenses? That's right, you!

Except in special situations, I see little need to buy a business from someone else. With the kind of technological and communications capabilities you now have at your disposal, the fact of the matter is that starting a new business has never been easier. The best rule of thumb to go by when starting your home-based business is to do what you love; the money will follow.

Step 2: Conduct Market Research

Major corporations spend millions of dollars determining the marketability of products and services before investing time and money. In order to determine whether or not your idea is a marketable one, you don't need to spend a lot of money. First, just use some common sense. Ask yourself the following questions:

- Is this a product or service people want and are currently using?

- Does my product or service make sense based on demographic and major economic trends?

- Does my product or service have certain "value added" advantages over the competition?

- Will enough people buy what I have at a price where I can make a profit?

- What is the profile of my typical client?

It's infinitely easier to market a product or service that is a variation of something that already exists, and one that people are using and paying real money for, than to invent something brand new. Of course, inventing a blockbuster new product can be lucrative, but I see little reason to go through all the time and expense that inventing something new requires. In terms of your actual research, I suggest asking people you know general questions about how they feel about your product or service. You don't need to tell them just yet that you are starting a new venture; you are simply seeking unbiased information from consumers as to whether they would buy something and, if so, at what price. You can accomplish your goal of a home-based business with much less time and money involved if you simply engage yourself in a field that you enjoy and that enough real people will pay enough real money so you can make a profit. Of course, with all the money you will save by working from home, you will get to enjoy more of your profits!

Step 3: Determine Your Costs

Who wants to be on a budget? The answer is, nobody. Budgets imply limitations and restricted freedom to use our money as we desire. I don't want you to begin your new venture with limited thinking, because it is your thinking that will ultimately create your success. That being said, as you begin your new home-based business venture, you will have to be very conscious of your start-up costs. These expenses are really your initial investment in your business and include office equipment, furniture, utilities, office supplies, advertising, travel, and professional fees such as accounting or legal charges. Make sure you have enough money to cover expenses until your new venture starts generating income. If you don't have the money on hand, you may want to look into a home equity loan, in which the interest is tax-deductible. Here are some good home equity loan Web sites to research:

HOME EQUITY LOAN WEB SITES

- E-Loan.com
- Countrywide.com
- Lendingtree.com
- Bankrate.com

Step 4: Develop Your Client Base

Vilfredo Pareto was an Italian economist of the late 1800s and early 1900s. He is best remembered for his observation that 20% of the people are responsible for 80% of the results. This is known as Pareto's Principle or the 80:20 Rule. As you begin your new business venture, keep Pareto's Principle in mind. Just 20% of your clients will ultimately account for 80% of your business. Therefore, you will need to quickly identify your primary target market—those people who best fit the profile of consumers of your product. You will then design your marketing and promotion around them. This will allow for the most efficient use of your time, money, and energy.

THE WORLD'S BEST ADVERTISING

There is an unlimited number of ways that you can develop an advertising campaign to kick-start your new business. The most effective advertising by far is word-of-mouth—the advertising your clients do for you because they have had a positive experience with your product or service. When you are first starting out, you don't have many clients; but don't let that stop you. If you are in a product-oriented business, be prepared to give away some free samples of your product and conduct free product demonstrations. With all the fantastic technology that we have at our fingertips today, one fact remains constant: there is nothing like meeting with people face to face. If you are in a service-oriented business, you are basically promoting yourself, so it is even more important for people to see you and get an up-close and personal idea of what you are like and how they might benefit from working with you. Get creative—go out to see the people!

As in any relationship, communication is key. You will want to communicate to your clientele and prospects regularly using regular mail, phone, e-mail, and personal contact. Of course, concentrate the majority of your resources on the best 20% of your clients. When you do, it's a win-win situation for you and your clients. Your best customers deserve most of your attention They are also the people who will most appreciate your services and tell their friends about you.

Step 5: The Magic Ingredient

If you have a product or a service that is superior or can provide people with something they can't quite get anywhere else, your chances of succeeding are very good. That being said, I must add that you will need to use all of the Key Principles of Success I provided in Chapter 1 in order to maximize your chances for success. These principles are crucial, particularly at the beginning stages of your business when you are still building the "critical mass"—the client base that will form the foundation of your business enterprise. I suggest that you read these principles every night before you go to sleep until they are firmly embedded in your subconscious. This will expedite the journey to your ultimate goal.

The magic ingredient in any venture you undertake is the person you look at in the mirror every day. You and you alone hold the key to your success. Just think about it for a second. What type of people do you like doing business with? When you are in the market for a particular product or service and the person advising you provides knowledgeable, unbiased advice and communicates clearly, aren't you very happy you have found that person? And isn't it a pretty safe bet he or she will keep your business? Sure it is. The idea is to just be the person you would like to do business with and—most importantly—be yourself at all times! As an example, if you have a natural sense of humor in business then use it, but if you are more the serious, get-to-the-point type, be yourself and don't try to emulate the person who uses humor. Regardless of your personality type, it's a good idea to keep in mind something said by Jay Leno on "The Tonight Show": "You can't stay mad at somebody who makes you laugh."

Just like you, successful people in this day and age have a very limited amount of time. When you help them quickly and efficiently, you are telling them that you respect their time. That, in turn tells them that you respect them as a person. By doing this you have just created a fantastic bond between you and one of your valued clients.

—*A Passion Play*—

Above all, your home-based business or home-based network marketing business should be a passionate experience for you and for those you communicate and work with. Find a product or service that really turns you on, that makes you feel energized and excited to begin your day (or evening, if you prefer). Your business should enhance your entire life, make your relationships with friends and family more fulfilling, and provide you with greater personal growth, achievement, and happiness. Be passionate and excited about what you do and everything else in your life will become better. Think big, set challenging goals, have total confidence in yourself, and always remember that your possibilities are only limited by the limits you place upon yourself by your thoughts. Congratulations on your decision to create a better way of life for yourself and everyone you know!

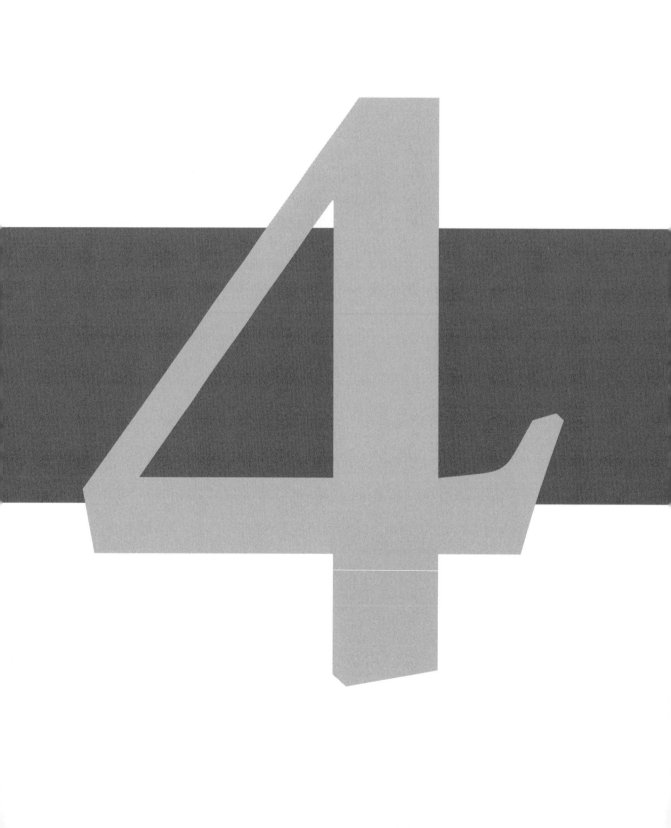

CHAPTER FOUR

Investing for Your Future

Investing for Your Future

**The greatest opportunity lies
at the point of maximum pessimism.**

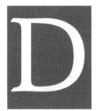uring the first several years of the 21st century investors endured a severe bear market for stocks, terrible acts of terrorism, and various corporate-related scandals. However, we Americans are an extremely resilient group of patriots, and, in the long run, our financial markets will prove equally resilient. Make no mistake about it, America's passion for investing is alive and well, and this passion to invest is sure to continue in many other parts of the world.

It seems as if, everywhere we turn today, someone has investment advice or an opinion on the stock market, retirement planning, IRAs, the economy, or even a new "hot" stock tip. The Internet has further fueled interest in global markets by making widely available the financial and investment information that once only professionals could access. Investing on-line has also played a major role in the long-term interest and participation of consumers in the financial markets. Here are some things you need to know as you prepare to invest:

—Stocks—

The stock of a corporation is simply an ownership position in that company. For instance, if you owned 1,000 shares of Microsoft you would actually own part of Microsoft, but a very small percentage of the corporation as a whole. There are thousands of stocks to choose from.

Stocks generally fall into one of two basic categories: *growth* or *value*. Growth stock investors are generally more aggressive; they pay greater attention to share price momentum and are willing to take on greater risk. Value investors, on the other hand, concern themselves more with something called a "price to earnings ratio" (P/E ratio). The P/E ratio is a stock valuation measurement that compares the earnings of a company to its stock price. In general, the lower the P/E ratio is, the greater the "value" investors are receiving for their money.

Selecting individual stocks to include in your portfolio is a serious matter. Done correctly, it is a time-consuming task involving considerable research. However, a vast amount of necessary information is available today; and if you wish to invest the time to do adequate research, stock-picking can be a rewarding experience.

Before you log on to your Internet provider and begin to conduct your research or possibly even invest on-line, let's take a step back and review some basic investing principles.

Five Basic Principles for Selecting Stocks

1. It's your money.

You are ultimately accountable for your stock portfolio. While stockbrokers, financial planners, Internet Web sites, and stock-savvy "experts" may provide seemingly fabulous ideas about what you should own, it's your money, and you must be willing to live with the decisions you make. You are ultimately responsible and no one else, so be well prepared before you invest!

2. Research before you invest.

I have always been amazed at how many people are willing to invest in a hot stock tip suggested by a friend, relative, or even a complete stranger at a cocktail party! There is a vast amount of stock research information available to you today in a split second on the Internet. Regardless of who makes a stock recommendation to you, first do your homework!

3. Your investments should be "tailor-made."

You are a unique individual with a personality, risk tolerance, goals, and a lifestyle all your own. Your investments should reflect your individuality. Your investments should never be chosen based on some mathematical formula that attempts to fit you into a category, especially as determined by your age. For example, don't think that, because you are over 60 or 70 years of age, you must have a certain percentage of your assets in stocks. The over-85 age group is currently the fastest growing segment of the U.S. population. This means that, if you are in your 60s or 70s, there's a very good chance that you may live past 85. This holds particularly true for women; according to U.S. Census Bureau's statistics, at age 85 women outnumber men five to two!

4. Be diversified.

Simply put, don't put all your eggs in one basket. One of the biggest mistakes an investor can make when designing a stock portfolio is to concentrate on too few stocks in too few market sectors. This is one disadvantage of choosing stocks over mutual funds. Diversifying an all-stock portfolio means that you select enough stocks in a variety of industry sectors (such as finance, technology, or health care) to achieve adequate asset allocation in your stock portfolio. Asset allocation is an investment technique whereby you diversify a certain percentage of your portfolio to different classes of assets, such as stocks, bonds, and cash. You therefore are faced with two allocation issues: one is choosing an adequate number of stocks in each sector; the other is invest in an adequate number of sectors.

The bottom line is that putting together a fully diversified portfolio of stocks can be very expensive when you consider trading fees and other expenses; in addition, it can consume a lot of your time! Buying stock mutual funds instead will allow you to concentrate more on industry sector selection and leave the actual choice of stocks up to the professionals.

5. Become a student of the stock market.

One of the difficult lessons of the stock market meltdown of the early 2000s is that, *in the long run,* stock prices are driven by profits, not by investor mania in "hot" stocks. When investors—particularly inexperienced investors—pour money into stocks simply because those stocks are appreciating in price, you have the makings of a stock market bubble. When the "Internet stock" bubble burst in 2000, the lesson was learned once again. Yes, you can earn short-term profits if you can get out in time, but then it's not really investing, it's more like casino gambling.

In the long run, the stock market is a great way to invest. The number of technological inventions will keep growing, and the solid companies that provide the infrastructure will continue to prosper. However, always be prepared for dramatic price volatility that can occur in the short-run, and never put into growth stocks the money that you will need for expenses in the near future.

I suggest educating yourself as much as you can about the stock market so that your expectations come as close as possible to your results. There are a variety of ways that you can teach yourself about the stock market. Visiting the investment section of your local public library or bookstore is a good way to start. You can also enroll in a course at a local college or even attend financial seminars conducted by investment professionals. Subscribing to the *Wall Street Journal* is also an excellent idea. Web sites such as www.smartmoney.com and www.bloomberg.com post interesting and informative articles on the stock market.

—*Mutual Funds*—

Today there are almost 9,000 mutual funds to choose from. In the past decade the mutual fund industry has experienced explosive growth, even with the market downturn of the early 2000s. In fact, the majority of mutual funds assets have appeared since 1991. Approximately $6.3 trillion is currently invested in mutual funds, up from $1.4 trillion in 1991 (Investment Company Institute, 2003).

What Is a Mutual Fund?

A mutual fund is an investment company that pools the money it receives from investors. That money is then invested based on the goal of the fund, which must be stated in the fund's prospectus. (A prospectus is document that the government requires mutual funds to provide. The prospectus explains important information about the fund, including its goals, risk level, and management fees.) Mutual funds provide investors with several major advantages over purchasing single stocks, including instant diversification, convenience, and the same professional management whether you have $1,000 or $1,000,000 invested in the fund. Mutual funds have various investment goals, but they may also have certain similarities to each other. For instance, some mutual funds seek to achieve "long-term growth" while others hope to provide you with "income and capital preservation." If you are seeking long-term growth of your investments, you would be a likely candidate for buying a *growth mutual fund* because these funds invest primarily in stocks that have provided average annual returns of over 10% since 1926 (source: Ibbotson Associates). Growth funds will generally have a greater degree of risk and a greater probability of better long-term performance than *income funds,* which concentrate on providing investors with income primarily through bonds and are less risky than growth funds because most bonds do not experience the big ups and down of stocks. (Investment risk refers to the price volatility of a particular investment as well as the potential for investment loss.) Also very popular are *growth and income* or *balanced* funds, which are a cross between growth funds and income funds.

Now it's time to determine which types of mutual funds are most appropriate for your investment portfolio.

Which Type of Fund Is Right for You?

With thousands of mutual funds and mutual fund managers in existence, mutual funds offer something for virtually everyone. Here's a look at the various classifications of mutual funds:

Sector Funds

Sector Funds invest in stock within a specific industry, such as health care, technology, energy, consumer industries and financial services. Sector funds allow you the opportunity to choose the market sectors that best suit your financial goals. Adding sector funds to your portfolio increases your risk (volatility) as well as your potential return because you are concentrating a greater percentage of your portfolio in one industry sector. Therefore, sector funds are generally more appropriate for investors who are willing to assume some degree of greater of risk for the potential for greater returns. In addition, sector funds are more suited to experienced investors who also may be knowledgeable about a specific industry sector. I urge you to use caution when selecting sector funds since you may experience more portfolio volatility than you are accustomed to. However, a prudent approach to sector fund selection can have its rewards.

Asset Allocation Funds

Also referred to as "flexible portfolio funds," *asset allocation funds* invest in a variety of different asset classes, such as stocks, bonds, money market, real estate, and precious metals. The fund manager determines the diversification of each of the classes within the fund. Asset allocation funds are good if you like the idea of the fund manager making all the decisions. These funds are typically suited to more conservative investors; but if you are interested in such a fund, be sure to carefully examine the fund's goals and objectives as described in its prospectus.

International Funds

If you like the idea of investing in Europe, Asia, Latin America, or anywhere else in the world besides the United States, you should examine *international mutual funds.* These funds are typically riskier than U.S. funds and don't always reward you monetarily for their increased volatility. However, with two-thirds of the world's investments outside of the U.S., international funds offer the promise of increased portfolio diversification with at least a potential for increased returns. *Proceed with caution.* Besides being riskier, international funds tend to be priced much higher than U.S. funds. While researching international funds, you may also come across the term *global mutual funds.* These funds invest both in the U.S. and abroad; international funds invest strictly outside the U.S.

Index Funds

If you like the idea of mutual funds managed primarily by a computer, *index funds* are for you. Index funds simply aim to match the composition and performance of investments in the index they represent. A *stock market index* is a group of stocks that provide a gauge of how a particular part of the stock market is performing. For example, the largest and best-known index fund, Vanguard's Index Trust 500 Fund, invests in the 500 stocks that make up the Standard and Poor's 500 Index. Usually referred to as the S&P 500, this index is a list of stocks of the 500 largest U.S. corporations. In a bull market or rising stock market, stock index funds tend to perform well because virtually all of the fund's money is invested all of the time, based on the guidelines set forth by the index and the fund's objectives. Of course, in a bear market or falling stock market, index funds have no safety net whatsoever because the fund simply cannot move into safer money market instruments or bonds.

Bond Funds

If you are seeking income instead of—or in addition to—growth, you will probably want to look at *bond mutual funds.* Like individual bonds, bond mutual funds represent debt issued by corporations, municipalities, federal agencies, and other governmental organizations.

A major difference between individual bonds and bond funds is that individual bonds have set interest rates and fixed maturity dates, whereas bond funds do not. Bond funds can have above-average risk—for example, high-yield bonds affectionately referred to as "junk bonds" in the 1980s. The same types of bonds exist today, only now they carry the "high yield" label, undoubtedly because the fund companies that promote them think "high-yield" sounds more appealing than "junk". However, bond funds come in other varieties, including corporate, government (including U.S. treasury bonds), tax-free (municipal), and international bond funds. In determining which bond fund is best for you, be sure to evaluate the quality of the bonds, interest rate, bond maturities, and bond fund taxation. A great deal of bond fund information can be found on the Web at www.morningstar.com. And of course, before investing your money, *always* review the fund's prospectus to determine the fund's management objectives and expenses.

Open-End Mutual Funds

This type of fund can accept an unlimited number of shareholders and cash. It is the kind of fund you normally see listed in the mutual fund section of your local paper. However, some open-end funds do close themselves to new investors after reaching a certain asset-size, out of concern for becoming too large and unmanageable. In this book, most of the discussion pertaining to mutual funds will be referring to open-end mutual funds.

Closed-End Mutual Funds

This type of fund issues a fixed number of shares when starting up. After that, the fund is traded just like a stock on a stock exchange and brokerage commissions are involved when you buy or sell closed-end funds. Stockbrokers tend to like closed-end funds since a sales commission is charged both when you buy a closed-end fund and when you sell it. Closed-end funds are a win-win situation for the stockbroker, but you should use an extra dash of common sense if a closed-end fund is offered to you.

Your Cost of Ownership

Determining what your mutual fund will cost has become more complicated. Just a short time ago you could have narrowed your choice to *load* mutual funds or *no-load* mutual funds. Mutual funds with loads had sales charges. No-load funds didn't have sales charges. It was like choosing between vanilla and chocolate ice cream. As with ice cream flavors, the choice of mutual funds is now virtually limitless. While load funds still have sales charges, remember that, like most things in life, investments are never completely "free." You will pay for your investment one way or another, sooner or later.

Load funds now allow you the choice between an *up-front load,* where you pay when you buy in, or a *back-end load,* also known as a *contingent deferred sales charge* (CDSC), where you pay a sales charge only if you redeem your fund within a certain period of time. Many funds now offer back-end loads with a charge as low as 1%. If you hold the fund for just one year, the back-end load is removed. The day of the pure no-load/no-fee fund family is nearing an end. As the costs of doing business rise, many no-load fund companies are able to maintain their no-load status only by charging you fees in other less obvious ways. Some no-load fund companies now charge redemption fees on certain funds in their fund family—often their bestselling funds. Some historically no-load fund families also offer low-load funds with up-front loads in the 1%–3% range. In addition, some no-load funds now charge something called *12b-1 fees,* which exist to reimburse the company for marketing and distribution costs. Previously, 12b-1 fees were associated only with loaded funds. The biggest drawback of the no-load fund family is that you receive little or no help managing your mutual fund portfolio. A trusted, unbiased professional advisor can be a valuable ally.

Choosing which mutual funds to buy is no longer a question of load versus no-load. It is a personal decision you must make based on your own financial goals and circumstances. It is of vital importance to educate yourself on the advantages and disadvantages of each type of mutual fund. Take it from someone who has spent thousands of hours over many years researching mutual funds: properly evaluating and selecting mutual funds is not a simple task. Once again, do your homework!

Consider some of the important factors involved when evaluating a mutual fund:

- Track record of fund family
- Performance in bear markets
- Risk as measured by the fund's beta
- Quality of management and tenure of fund's manager
- Securities that make up the fund
- Expenses (loads, redemption fees, 12b-1 fees, etc.)
- Interest and dividend yields
- Ratings by independent fund data providers
- Percentage of securities in each market sector
- Expected impact inflation will have on your fund
- Tax-efficiency rating
- Retirement vs. nonqualified account
- Index fund vs. managed fund
- Concentration or diversification of fund
- Asset allocation decisions

With the vast amount of information available to most people today from books, newspapers, magazines, satellite and cable TV, and the Internet, it's easy enough to get plenty of information. But remember that the media's ultimate goal is to have you tune in so that they can sell more advertising space at a greater profit; don't ever lose sight of this motive. So much of the information we are exposed to is just noise—that is, information sensationalized to attract the listener (or viewer) and designed to sell information for the benefit of the information provider but not necessarily the information recipient.

—Asset Allocation: Making Smart Investment Choices—

Call it *diversification, asset allocation,* or simply "not putting all your eggs in one basket"— it all means the same thing. Smart investing involves not only choosing the right investments but also devising the proper combination of investments. Otherwise, you run the risk of having too much money concentrated in one particular type of investment; and if its value should decline greatly, so does your financial status. This principal applies to stocks, mutual funds, and virtually every other type of investment.

What is and what isn't diversification? Owning ten different pieces of real estate is *not* an example of diversification. Owning ten different mutual funds or ten different stocks doesn't guarantee diversification either. Proper investment diversification involves a variety of factors that in most cases require a great deal of know-how or help from an investment professional to figure out. There is a vast universe of investment choices today. Achieving sound diversification in your portfolio involves selecting the right balance of investments so that your dollars are spread across a variety of investments.

The Investment Pyramid

The investment pyramid on page 107 illustrates the concept of investment risk and return regarding asset allocation. The base of the pyramid represents a relatively low level of return and a high degree of predictability. Risk and the potential for better performance (greater yield) both increase as you work your way up the pyramid. For instance, futures contracts, options contracts, and speculative common stocks and bonds have relatively high risk but potentially higher returns. Conversely, money market accounts, treasury securities, and U.S. savings bonds have very low risk, along with the probability of lower long-term returns than many other investment choices. Use the investment pyramid as a guide when mapping out your personal asset allocation strategy. As you design your asset allocation strategy, refer to this investment pyramid to gauge your degree of investment risk.

The hot stock tip of the day may make you some quick money in the short run *if you are lucky,* but your investment planning will be very difficult and highly speculative. Don't rely on the hot stock tip or luck when designing your investment plan. Instead, rely on extensive research and solid investment choices.

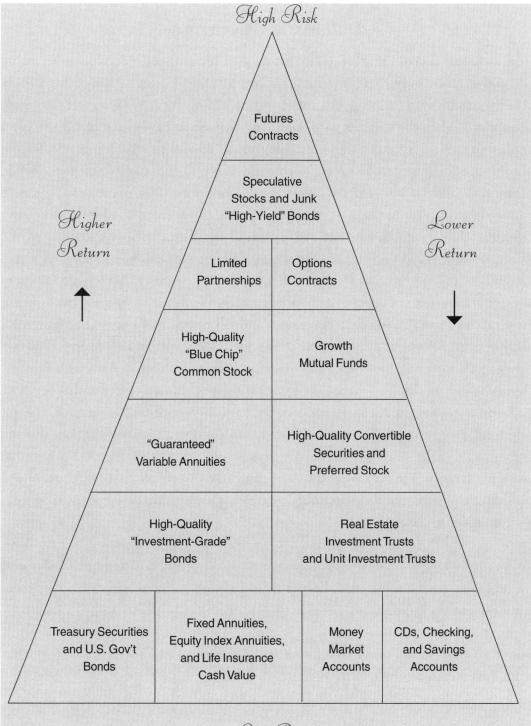

—*Dollar Cost Averaging*—

Human nature dictates that, when investing your own money, you will be driven by two powerful and overwhelming emotions: fear and greed. I am certain of this, having observed a variety of investors of all ages and from all walks of life who were in a state of euphoria when the markets were going up and somewhere between nervous and panic-stricken when the markets were going down. You know what it's like: When the markets are going up, you're saying to yourself, "I wish I had invested more money in the market." Even if you've never invested a penny before, if the markets are going up you wished you had started! Conversely, when the markets are headed down, you're thinking "How soon can I get my money out of the market before I lose my shirt!" That's called the fight-or-flight response, something that has been genetically programmed into the human brain over the ages. So, do you really think you're going to overcome thousands of years of gene-pool evolution by training yourself to automatically refrain from flinching during a stock market plunge? Of course not; but don't despair, because there is a proven investment technique that can help keep you calmly invested during good times and bad. This technique is called *dollar cost averaging.* Here's how it works: You invest the same amount of money each month—let's say $500—in a mutual fund, consistently, every month without fail. Over time, market prices will go up and market prices will go down. What you are counting on is that the overall trend of the stock market will be positive in the long run. During the past 200 years the trend of the stock market has been generally positive, although extended periods of market downturns have occurred. Be vigilant in educating yourself on market conditions and trends.

While dollar cost averaging cannot guarantee you a profit, a disciplined dollar cost averaging program has proven to be one of the simplest and most effective investment strategies ever developed.

The table on page 109 provides a hypothetical illustration of how a dollar cost averaging plan could work:

DOLLAR COST AVERAGING EXAMPLE

Invested Each Quarter	Price per Share	Number of Shares
$1,000	$50	20
$1000	$50	20
$1000	$40	25
$1000	$25	40
$1000	$25	40
$1000	$40	25
$1000	$50	20
Total Amount Invested: $7000	Average Price per Share: $40	Total Shares = 190 Average Cost per Share: $36.84 Savings per Share: $3.16

In this example you would have paid an average of $36.84 per share for the fund. That is better than the $50 per share you would have paid if you had instead invested all your money as a lump sum in the first quarter (see chart), but not so good as if you had lump-summed at $25 per share in quarter four.

While there is no perfect investment system, dollar cost averaging does offer you a prudent way to reduce the emotional roller coaster ride you might otherwise experience when investing in the stock market. You reduce the temptation of investing at market peaks, when your greed instinct is activated, and also reduce the temptation to pull your investments out of the stock market during "corrections" (market downturns) when your fear instinct tries to take control. In essence, you won't make the classic mistake of trying to "time the market."

Dollar cost averaging offers another major benefit: you will be less tempted to invest in the hot stock tip of the day. Investing in the stock market is a long-term proposition and should be approached with a steady mind. Always keep in mind the age-old saying that, "If it sounds too good to be true, it probably is."

Certainly, the most important thing for you to remember about dollar cost averaging is that, when it is done correctly, it will allow you to keep your investment dollars working 100% of the time toward the accomplishment of your financial goals.

For the vast majority of people, lasting financial success will not come free or easily. Unfortunately, many investors find out the hard way by losing money and precious time before coming to this simple conclusion. Mutual fund investing is all about determining your goals, researching your alternatives, and putting together an asset allocation strategy to accomplish those goals. Mutual fund investing is inherently long-term in nature. Your investment and learning experience with mutual funds can and should be a positive and rewarding experience as well.

—*Exchange Traded Funds*—

An alternative to both mutual funds and stocks that deserves your consideration is something called *exchange traded funds* (ETFs). These funds are actually a cross between stocks and mutual funds and are listed on the American Stock Exchange and New York Stock Exchange. With ETFs you can buy a complete portfolio of stocks in one single security. ETFs are available that invest in the broad market, market sectors, or international indices. Here are some of the most popular ETFs:

- Diamonds (symbol: DIA), which invests in the 30 stocks that make up the Dow Jones Industrial Average

- SPDRs (symbol: SPY), which invest in the S&P 500

- The Nasdaq 100 Index Tracking Stock (symbol QQQ), which includes the 100 largest nonfinancial stocks on the NASDAQ

ETFs have some very desirable benefits:

- A complete portfolio of stocks in one security

- Ability to buy or sell during the trading day unlike mutual funds

- Much easier portfolio diversification and tracking than individual stocks

- Eligible for margin buying and IRAs

- Invest in an entire portfolio of stocks more economically and quickly than with individual stocks

- No management fees (not like mutual funds)

If you are a stock market investor and haven't considered ETFs before, take a closer look; you just might like what you see.

CHAPTER FIVE

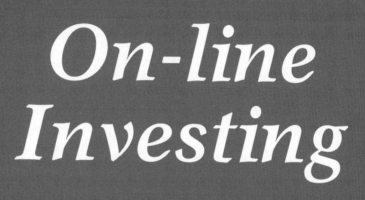

On-line Investing

On-line Investing

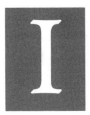

I t wasn't too long ago that many scoffed at the idea of using the Internet as a place to research investments and as a place to invest your hard-earned money. While the economic downturn of the early 2000s and the impact of terrorism had a negative effect on the short-term growth of on-line investing, prospects for future growth are still very good.

While the long-term growth of on-line investing looks promising, it is also true that not everyone wants to spend the many hours it takes to conduct effective investment research on-line. Scores of investors learned the hard way during the market downturn and economic recession of the early 2000s, particularly those investors who found it "oh so easy" to buy high-flying technology stocks with the click of a computer mouse. As we found out later, many of those high-flying technology stocks crashed to the ground, taking investors' money right along with them.

Stories of business executives losing their multi-million-dollar pensions and housewives wiping out the children's college tuition via day trading are not only true, they're downright terrifying.

The Council on Compulsive Gambling in New Jersey estimates that 5% of all day traders are addicted gamblers who aren't in it for anything but the thrills. Some of these "addicted" traders use equity lines of credit on their homes and cash advances on credit cards to buy stock on-line. Their uncontrolled addictions can have dire financial consequences for themselves and their families. Day trading is very serious business and should always be undertaken with a reasonable and rational mindset.

—On-line Research—

If you are going to begin investigating whether you should even consider do-it-yourself on-line investing, first do some extensive fundamental research. Here are some of the Web sites you should explore:

- Bigcharts.com
- Investor.com
- Morningstar.com
- Smartmoney.com
- Bloomberg.com
- Mfcafe.com
- Nasdaqtrader.com
- Zacks.com

While checking these out will start you off on the right foot, there is a major difference between browsing research Web sites on-line and actually investing your hard-earned retirement assets with a quick click of your mouse. One major financial mistake could, of course, cost you your lifestyle of choice in retirement, a new home, or any other financial goal. The decision to be your own investment manager is a very serious move; to be successful, you will need to spend a great deal of time and acquire a great deal of expertise.

Before determining whether you should do your own investing on-line or hire a financial professional, weigh the pros and cons of both alternatives.

—The Advantages of On-line Investing—

1. Lower expenses

If you can master the art of investing on your own, the on-line approach is your cheapest route, from the standpoint of fees and costs. The major reason is that there is no professional advice provided and therefore no charges except trading fees. As usual, you get what you pay for here; and, as many investors have learned, saving yourself from making one major financial mistake may justify hiring professional help.

2. Control over trade execution

When you trade on-line, your computer (and mouse) complete the trade. There is no need for a phone call to your broker or financial planner. You're in complete control. Remember that also means that you must confirm trade execution. I urge you to make a regular habit of confirming with your on-line broker that your trade has been made. Mistakes can happen when you place a trade on-line, especially on days with high trading volume in the stock market.

3. No human interaction

If you're a true do-it-yourselfer, on-line investing will appeal to you. But if you become uneasy or want some prudent and personal financial advice, don't expect to find a knowledgeable human on the Web site for free. In times of heavy trading volume, not being able to access competent help immediately can be a particularly troublesome problem. Some on-line trading firms offer financial advice, however, as with any other type of professional advice, you will be paying for it one way or another.

4. You're the boss

When you trade on-line, you call all the shots. You determine what to invest in and when. It's you and your computer managing your financial future. If you are willing to invest many hours in research and learn the dynamics of on-line trading, then this may be the investing style for you.

—The Advantages of Hiring a Financial Professional—

1. Experienced, knowledgeable, and unbiased advice

When you work with a trained investment professional, you are getting someone who should be able to help you avoid major financial mistakes while assisting you in achieving your financial goals. Furthermore, if you're working with an unbiased professional who has no proprietary (in-house) products to sell, that person has your best interests in mind and, above all else, wants you to succeed. Be cautious with financial planners and stockbrokers who are promoting mutual funds, annuities, insurance, or other investments that bear the same name as their company. They may be recommending them to you because selling those financial products will bring them substantially larger commissions. To be sure that you are getting objective, unbiased advice, seek out financial advisors who do not have proprietary or company-owned products to sell.

2. Communication and goal setting

You can communicate to a qualified professional financial advisor everything you want to achieve with your investments. Based on your goals, the advisor can develop a plan to help you achieve the lifestyle you desire. While some people may choose to do their financial planning on-line, others will prefer dealing with a human being.

3. Help in a bear market

Many of the on-line traders who thought of themselves as stock market geniuses during the high-flying 1990s began seeking good advice during the troubled markets of the early 2000s. Having someone trustworthy to confide in when times get tough can give you priceless peace of mind.

4. Less frantic trading

On-line trading tends to promote just that—a lot of "trading." Even with inexpensive trades, costs do add up over time when you're placing lots of trades. Keep in mind that, when you make a profitable trade, the IRS wants their piece of the action, too. A good financial professional can teach you the value of investing in quality securities and fine-tuning your investing program only when it's necessary, which in the long run will save you money.

5. Complete financial advice

A really good financial advisor should know more about financial matters than just how to choose and buy stocks. You should be able to talk to your advisor about any financial move you are considering, such as refinancing a mortgage, leasing versus buying your auto, ways to reduce income and estate taxes, decisions regarding IRAs and 401(k) plans, even health and long-term care insurance issues. Your advisor may even be able to advise you on starting a business of your own.

6. A caring human being

We all know how frustrating it can be looking for a knowledgeable and courteous person to talk with these days. This applies not only to financial advice, but to any service you seek. It seems as if almost every company is trying to cut costs, and that generally results in your having to talk to someone's voice mail or communicating by e-mail. While the Internet is a fabulous and revolutionary information resource,

I don't think it will ever completely replace talking to a human being who sincerely cares about you, particularly when the conversation is about your money.

—*The Bottom Line*—

When you are considering an investment, examine all the costs involved, but pay closest attention to how much net profit you are making. In figuring your profits you should take into consideration tax savings, guarantees, asset appreciation, dividends and interest, and how much gain you actually "lock in." As many investors who participated in the Internet bubble discovered, it's not how much profit you have on paper that counts, but rather how much profit you can ultimately turn into guaranteed income or cash. Many experienced financial advisors who were charging hefty management and/or financial planning fees of up to 3% of your assets per year in the go-go 1990s will now waive your out-of-pocket fees if you place your assets under their management. Always seek out an unbiased advisor with no proprietary (in-house) products, which ultimately taint the client-advisor relationship. While no professional can infallibly predict the future performance of your investments (with the exception of some annuities that are guaranteed by the issuer), it's your bottom line that counts the most.

As we progress further into the age of the Internet, it is quite likely that many investors will want the best of both worlds: the ability to access the Internet for investing and research as well as quick access to the trustworthy advice of a caring, knowledgeable financial professional. What most people really care about is not making a permanent choice between a computer and a human being, but achieving their desired lifestyle.

Utilizing Internet technology along with the assistance of your chosen financial advisor will give you your best chance to live the lifestyle you desire for as long as you live. As communications and information technologies evolve and expand, talking with your financial advisor no longer means that you must be inhabiting the same physical space. Today, video conferencing, cell phones, and communicating via satellite and the wireless Internet will allow you to easily connect with your financial advisor from anywhere in the world at any time. The costs for all of these communications services will decrease as the technologies continue to improve.

CHAPTER SIX

Your Retirement Lifestyle

Your Retirement Lifestyle

> ### *The best is yet to come!*

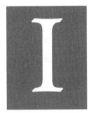n the 21st century, Americans will live much longer than in previous centuries. Today over 50,000 Americans, about one out of every 5,700, is 100 years of age or older. In 1950, only one out of every 30,000 Americans reached age 100. It is projected that by 2050, over 1,000,000 Americans will be age 100 or older. In addition, it is estimated that the 85-plus age group will quadruple in size from 1999 to 2040 (U.S. Census Bureau). According to Nationwide Life Insurance Company, of couples reaching age 65, there is a 94% chance one will live past 80 and a 63% chance of one living past 90.

Since there is a good chance that you (and your spouse, if you're married) will live longer than you ever imagined, your money will have to last longer, too. That means adopting a long-term view of your finances and developing investing strategies. One of the biggest mistakes people make while planning for retirement is underestimating how long they will live.

—Digital Age Economics 101: Inflation Meets Deflation—

The Digital Age has brought about a multitude of economic changes. One of the most unusual and important developments is that, in the age of the Internet, we have both inflationary and deflationary forces to contend with simultaneously.

Increased global competition is a byproduct of the information explosion we are now experiencing. More and more goods bought in the U.S. are made overseas, in places such as China and India, where labor costs are much lower. Products that can be made in one part of the world and purchased elsewhere result in a downward spiral of prices, otherwise known as deflation. The ability to search for the best price, then make the purchase over the Internet, further fuels deflation. Some examples of goods involved in this "spiral effect" are computers, furniture, and clothing. According to a study by the American Textile Manufacturers Institute, China could control up to 75% of the U.S. textile and apparel market by 2005 ("The Journal of Commerce," 7/7/03). Another example of the effect of low labor costs is that television sets have become so inexpensive to build in Asia that some companies now offer free TVs as buying inducements much as banks used to give away free toasters to those who opened new accounts.

The reality is that the effect of the Internet is inherently deflationary. Computers and electronics are not the only products affected; other goods include clothing, furniture, airline tickets, and some automobiles. A deflationary spiral causes intense price competition, making it very difficult for companies to raise prices. This condition leads to a weak economy, layoffs in the workforce, and elimination of production facilities due to weak demand. Acquisition of new capital equipment is delayed, causing a domino effect.

The only way corporations can improve their bottom line in this scenario is by cost-cutting, which does not help to create growth in the economy or in the job market. One of the positive aspects of deflation is lower interest rates, resulting in very attractive mortgage rates in recent years. Lower mortgage interest rates have been the primary driver in the escalation of U.S. real estate prices. If economic conditions worsen or become stagnant, real estate prices could fall even if interest rates remain low by historical standards. The reality will always be that real estate is only worth what someone is willing to pay for it.

At the opposite end of the economic spectrum in the Digital Age is inflation, which means price appreciation. Before the U.S. received its first real dose of deflation since the great depression, inflation was seen as the predominant economic threat.

While the type of runaway inflation we saw in the early 1980s is still seen as a threat, because of the ongoing threat of deflation, inflation is now viewed as necessary for economic growth.

Prices in certain sectors of the economy, especially those related to local services, have been escalating. Local services are not currently subjected in a major way to global competition (though global forces may ultimately force even local service costs down) and therefore tend to be inflationary. Good examples of price inflation include health care, college education, and insurance costs.

In the 20-year period from 1980 to 2000, health care costs rose 257%, a 12.85% average annual increase. From 2000 to 2003 health care costs have risen by a more moderate 8% per year (source: Kaiser Family Foundation). The average worker has seen a 26% rise in health-care insurance premiums since 2000.

The college tuition picture is also highly inflationary. A college student enrolling at Stanford University in 2000–2001 experienced a 17% increase in tuition by the 2003–2004 academic year, and Stanford is by no means the exception. Tuition and fees at private colleges have risen 18% since the 1999–2000 academic year.

Regarding insurance costs, from 2000 to 2003 homeowner's insurance rose an average of 6.4% per year, while auto insurance increased 7.6% per year (source: Insurance Information Institute).

The bottom line to this paradoxical economy that exhibits both deflationary and inflationary characteristics is that, on the whole, it is simply getting much more expensive to live. The rate of inflation (up 2.5% annually the past three years, as measured by the U.S. Bureau of Labor Statistics) clearly understates the increased real cost of living for the average American.

—*The Gold Watch: Industrial Age Museum Piece*—

The days of retiring at age 62 or 65 and depending on your Social Security check to carry you through retirement are quickly disappearing. Furthermore, the days of working for the same company for 30 years and retiring with the proverbial gold watch are also over. Maybe this worked well in the heyday of the Industrial Revolution or during the post-World War II era, but, like it or not, those days are long gone.

While today's economic realities may not have the predictable characteristics they did in days gone by, you have many excellent retirement investment choices today that were not previously available. It is up to you to choose the best retirement plan for your unique requirements, but I'll provide you with the information you'll need to make that decision.

Your retirement lifestyle can be whatever you want it to be, limited only by your imagination and by the steps you take and act upon to achieve it. Focus on designing your own unique and personal retirement investing strategy that will allow you to live the lifestyle you desire for as long as you live. Follow my four steps to retirement success to achieve your ultimate retirement lifestyle.

—*Four Steps to Retirement Success*—

Step 1: Evaluate Your Current Financial Position

The initial step toward achieving retirement success is to evaluate where you are today. You will need to perform two exercises. The first is to compare your income and your expenses. Income minus expenses is called *net income.* If your expenses are greater than your income, you could be heading into a dangerous financial situation, particularly with regards to your retirement planning. On page 127 I have provided an Income and Expenses Worksheet to help you calculate your net income.

If your expenses are higher than your income, do not despair. Instead, evaluate your expenses thoroughly to see if there are opportunities for cost cutting. In any event, take steps to lower your expenses, increase your income, or both.

CASH FLOW DATA—INCOME AND EXPENSES

ANNUAL INCOME

Employment/self-employment .... _____

Social Security .... _____

Investment income .... _____

Pensions.. _____

IRA distributions .... _____

Rental income/notes receivable .... _____

Other income .... _____

Total income .... $_____

ANNUAL EXPENSES

Mortgage payment #1 .... _____

Mortgage payment #2 .... _____

Real estate taxes .... _____

Utilities... _____

Homeowner's insurance .... _____

Home improvements .... _____

Food/personal care .... _____

Clothing/laundry/dry cleaning .... _____

Auto maintenance/insurance/license .... _____

Auto loan/lease .... _____

Medical/dental/prescriptions .... _____

Medical insurance premiums .... _____

Life insurance premiums .... _____

Nursing home insurance premiums .... _____

Entertainment/dining .... _____

Recreation/travel/hobbies .... _____

Education/subscriptons/gifts/misc... _____

Income taxes .... _____

Total Annual Expenses .... $_____

Total income .... $_____

Less Total Expenses .... $_____

ANNUAL DISCRETIONARY INCOME .... $_____

NET WORTH DATA—ASSETS AND LIABILITIES

ASSETS

Primary residence .... $\quad$ _____

Vacation/second residence .... _____

Home furnishings .... _____

Automobiles .... _____

Jewelry/art/furs/collectibles .... _____

Cash/checking/money market .... _____

Certificates of deposit .... _____

Stocks and stock mutual funds .... _____

Bonds and bond mutual funds .... _____

Tax-free bonds/funds .... _____

Life insurance cash value.. _____

Life insurance death benefit .... _____

Notes receivable .... _____

Limited partnership .... _____

IRA .... _____

Qualified plan (e.g. 401K) .... _____

Annuities (fixed or variable)... _____

Other assets .... _____

Total Assets .... $_____

LIABILITIES

Mortgage payment #1 .... _____

Mortgage payment #2 .... _____

Auto loans .... _____

Credit cards .... _____

Other liabilities .... _____

Total Liabilities .... $_____

Total Assets .... $_____

Less Total Expenses .... $_____

NET WORTH .... $_____

The second exercise is to evaluate your net worth. Here, you will compare your assets (the things you own) against your liabilities (what you owe). The amount of assets you have over and above your liabilities is called your *net worth.*

If your liabilities exceed your assets, this should be a signal to you that you should pay greater attention to building your assets for retirement. In order to do this you will either have to pay off some of your debt (liabilities) or increase your assets through savings, investments, or increased income. On page 128 you will find a Net Worth Statement Worksheet to help you evaluate your assets versus your liabilities.

Step 2: Set Your Retirement Goals

The next step of your journey toward achieving your desired retirement lifestyle is to write down your goals. Be as specific as you can. For this exercise, I suggest that you use index cards because they are small enough to fit in your day planner or purse and are more durable than paper. Write down the *specific* lifestyle you desire along with the amount of money you believe it will take to make it happen. An example of one person's retirement lifestyle goal is as follows: "I want to spend my retirement living in a beautiful home overlooking Lake Winnipesaukee, New Hampshire; purchase a new SUV; and take frequent vacations to the Caribbean and Europe. To achieve these goals I will earn $100,000 per year in retirement. My time frame for achieving my goal is 20 years." Remember, you are striving to achieve your own unique retirement goals, not someone else's. Write what your heart really desires.

Step 3: Do the Math

The next step is to calculate how much money it will take to get you from point A (where you are now) to point B (where you want to go). Many investors make a serious mistake here by underestimating how much money it will actually take to achieve their retirement goals. *Do not underestimate your projected expenses in retirement.* Make certain to consider costs such as long-term care insurance (or long-term care), inflation, taxes, travel, gifts, and home improvements. It is best to over-project—in other words, to overshoot your actual retirement income needs.

It is common to make the mistake of underestimating retirement expenses. At your retirement, wouldn't it be a nice surprise to find out you have *more* money than you had planned for? Sure it would. The earlier you begin planning, the easier this will be to achieve. If you have not begun planning for retirement as of today, start immediately!

Let's look at a simple example of how to calculate the amount of income you will need in retirement. Let's say that after careful consideration of your current and projected expenses, you decide you will need $100,000 of income in retirement to achieve the type of lifestyle you desire. If you could earn an 8% net return (after inflation and taxes) on your money, then $1,250,000 would be the amount of assets you would require to generate the $100,000 income ($1,250,000 x 8% = $100,000).

Now the challenge becomes "how do I determine how much I will need to invest during my retirement savings years to reach my ultimate goal?" To determine this number you will need to calculate how much you plan on saving per year and what rate of interest you expect to receive on your money. Again, taxes and inflation will have to be taken into consideration. You can perform these calculations on any good financial calculator or go to Quicken.com. or Smartmoney.com and access their retirement calculators 24 hours a day, seven days a week.

As an example, let's say again that you plan on amassing $1.25 million dollars for your retirement and you have 20 years to do so. If you didn't have any retirement savings today at all, it would take about $1,270 per month in savings at a 12% net rate of return (after inflation and taxes) to amass $1.25 million in 20 years. You can customize your plan with your tax bracket, estimated inflation rate, rates of investment return and so on. You could probably finish this exercise in about 10 minutes using one of the calculators. Since much of the calculations are based on assumed inflation rates and investment returns, always be conservative in your estimates in the event that the assumptions you made do not work out quite as well as you had hoped.

Step 4: Select the Best Investments to Reach Your Goal

Remember when there were only three flavors of ice cream: chocolate, vanilla and strawberry? Today you can choose from flavors like Superman Bubble Gum, Chunky Monkey, Cookie Dough Fantasia—a virtually limitless variety of flavors. The number of available choices with regard to your retirement investments has grown in a similar fashion. The days of defined pension plans, when workers could expect a certain amount of retirement income at a certain age, are now relics of the past for most people. While some do enjoy this predictable income from a bygone era, most people who are currently planning their ideal retirement lifestyle—and those who are already retired but want to establish a new retirement lifestyle—are faced with a dizzying array of choices. While the many investment "flavors" may seem daunting at first, once you have an understanding of the fundamentals of various retirement plans, you will feel much better and much more confident of your decision.

Let's take a look at some the retirement plans available to you. They are all considered *qualified* retirement plans—plans that receive favorable tax treatment from the Internal Revenue Service.

—*Qualified Retirement Plans*—

Traditional IRA

This is the original version of the popular retirement investment, also referred to as a "tax-deductible IRA" (Individual Retirement Account). All contributions to this type of IRA are deductible from your gross income for tax purposes. Traditional IRAs allow individuals with earned income to invest $3,000 per year in the form of a tax-deductible contribution. The annual IRA contribution limits have been increased by the federal government; the phased-in increases are as follows:

> 2003 through 2004: $3,000
>
> 2005 through 2007: $4,000
>
> 2008 and beyond: $5,000
>
> (From 2009 on, contribution limits will adjust annually for inflation in $500 increments.)

In addition, investors who are 50 years of age or older with earned income were allowed to contribute an additional $500 starting in 2002 and can contribute an additional $1,000 per year over the IRA contribution limits beginning in 2006.

All earnings inside the traditional IRA grow on a tax-deferred basis. That means there is no tax due until you withdraw money, and only the assets withdrawn are taxable. All contributions and earnings are taxed as ordinary income when withdrawn. Money you withdraw prior to reaching age 59½ may be subject to a 10% federal tax penalty.

Traditional IRA Limitations

Eligibility to deduct contributions from your taxes is phased out for active participants in employer-sponsored retirement plans such as 401(k) or 403(b) plans. In 2003, for example, the phase-out ranges for employer-sponsored retirement plans are $40,000 to $50,000 of *adjusted gross income* (AGI) for single persons and heads of households, $60,000 to $70,000 for married people filing jointly, and $0 to $10,000 for married people filing separately. Below are the phase-out ranges for 2004–2007:

Traditional IRA Deduction Phase-Out Ranges

	Single Taxpayer	Married Taxpayers Filing Jointly
2004	$45,000–55,000	$65,000–75,000
2005	$50,000–60,000	$70,000–80,000
2006	$50,000–60,000	$75,000–85,000
2007	$50,000–60,000	$80,000–100,000

For 2004–2007 phase-out ranges for married couples filing jointly is $0–$10,000. Also, if your spouse has an employer-sponsored retirement plan and you don't, your phase-out range is between $150,000 and $160,000.

Required Minimum Distributions

IRA participants *must* begin taking mandatory withdrawals (required minimum distributions) by April 1 of the year after they reach age 70½. The way the IRS figures it, you should now feel obligated to start paying tax on the built-up tax-deferred gains in your IRA. In fact, the government's budget depends on it. If you fail to make your *required minimum distribution* (RMD) at the prescribed time, the IRS will assess a 50% penalty on the amount you should have taken out of your IRA but did not. Under new IRS rules, your required minimum distribution is determined yearly by dividing your account balance on December 31st of the previous year by an age-based distribution period as shown in the table on page 133.

UNIFORM DISTRIBUTION TABLE

Age	Applicable Divisor	Age	Applicable Divisor
70	26.2	93	8.8
71	25.3	94	8.3
72	24.4	95	7.8
73	23.5	96	7.3
74	22.7	97	6.9
75	21.8	98	6.5
76	20.9	99	6.1
77	20.1	100	5.7
78	19.2	101	5.3
79	18.4	102	5.0
80	17.6	103	4.7
81	16.8	104	4.4
82	16.0	105	4.1
83	15.3	106	3.8
84	14.5	107	3.6
85	13.8	108	3.3
86	13.1	109	3.1
87	12.4	110	2.8
88	11.8	111	2.6
89	11.1	112	2.4
90	10.5	113	2.2
91	9.9	114	2.0
92	9.4	115 (and older)	1.8

As an example, let's say Helen, a hypothetical investor, has a traditional IRA account balance on December 31, 2003, of $600,000. In 2003, Helen will be 74 years old. According to the uniform distribution table (above), Helen's distribution period is 22.7 years. Therefore, Helen's minimum IRA distribution for 2003 would be $26,431 ($600,000 divided by 22.7). Helen must take her 2003 distribution by December 31,

2004. If she does not, the IRS will impose a whopping 50% penalty on the amount of Required Minimum Distributions that have not been taken.

Roth IRA

The Roth IRA was introduced in 1998. As with a traditional IRA, you may invest up to $3,000 per year beginning in 2002 if you are eligible. (Check the Roth IRA limitations for Eligibility Rules to determine your eligibility.) If you are eligible for a Roth IRA, I encourage you to invest in one. The Roth IRA has an overwhelming advantage over the traditional IRA: withdrawals from Roth IRAs after age 59½ are tax-free.

Besides untaxed growth, Roth IRAs offer another advantage; flexible withdrawal rules. You can withdraw contributions (not gains) for any reason at any time without penalties or taxes. After you reach age 59½, provided you have had your Roth IRA for five years, you may withdraw your gains, too, without any penalty tax. You may also withdraw your gains if you become disabled.

Roth IRA vs. Traditional IRA

Let's say, for example, that you have invested $3,000 per year for 15 years in both a Roth IRA and a traditional IRA. Assume that both investments grew at an average annual rate of return of 10%. After 15 years, assuming no withdrawals, each account would be worth $104,849. The big difference is that, with the traditional IRA, any money you withdraw is taxed as ordinary income, while your Roth IRA withdrawals are 100% tax-free. For instance, if you are in the 27% tax bracket and you withdraw $10,000 from your traditional IRA, you would be taxed $2,800. With your Roth IRA your tax is $0 (assuming you observe the Roth IRA withdrawal restrictions). Of course, this example does not consider the tax-deductibility of the traditional IRA, but even with that considered, for most people the Roth IRA is a superior investment.

Roth IRA Limitations

Not everyone is eligible to open a Roth IRA. If you are single with a *modified adjusted gross income* (MAGI) below $95,000 per year, you may contribute the full

$3,000 to a Roth IRA. This $3,000 limit begins to phase out as your income grows. Once your MAGI hits $110,000, you are no longer eligible for a Roth IRA. For married couples filing jointly, with a minimum MAGI of $150,000, you may contribute the full $3,000. At $160,000 you are no longer eligible. For married couples filing separately, the phase-out range is between $0 and $10,000.

Roth IRA Withdrawal Restrictions

Withdrawals from a Roth IRA are tax-free only if the Roth IRA owner has held the account for at least 5 years. In addition, the withdrawal must be made with at least one of the following additional conditions present:

> * Owner is age 59½ or older.
> * Owner is disabled.
> * Owner is deceased.
> * The money withdrawn will be used to pay up to $10,000 in first-time home-buying expenses.

SEP IRA

The Simplified Employee Pension (SEP) IRA is an excellent retirement plan for the self-employed. This plan offers an easy way to establish your retirement plan with no adoption or administration costs. Also, the IRS requires no annual reports as it does with some other qualified retirement plans. In figuring tax-deferred earnings and deductible contributions, the SEP IRA follows the same rules as a traditional IRA.

401(k) Plans

A 401(k) is a type of personal pension plan offered by your employer. It is without question one of the best retirement investment opportunities you will have in your lifetime. Here are some of the reasons why the 401(k) plan is one of the finest retirement savings plans available:

Pre-tax contributions: Contributions to your 401(k) plan are taken out of your paycheck before federal, state and local taxes are deducted, so this automatically lowers your income taxes. This is undoubtedly a marvelous technique to reduce your income taxes. Here are the maximum 401(k) contribution limits through 2006:

2002	$11,000
2003	$12,000
2004	$13,000
2005	$14,000
2006	$15,000

Tax-deferred earnings: Much as in a traditional IRA, your earnings in a 401(k) plan grow on a tax-deferred basis. This means that the IRS won't get any of it until you retire and begin withdrawing money.

Company match: Most employers offer to match a percentage or set dollar amount for every dollar you contribute. For instance, if your employer is matching your contribution by 50 cents on the dollar, you make an immediate 50% return on your money. With the pressures that have been placed on corporate profits and the resulting incrased use of technology and global workers to cut costs, many employers have reduced or eliminated matching 401(k) contributions altogether. If your employer is still offering a matching contribution, I suggest that you seriously consider taking it. This is an incredibly desirable feature, particularly considering the plight of many workers in the Digital Age.

Automatic payroll deduction: Putting your retirement savings plan on "autopilot" removes one of the most destructive psychological barriers to successful investing: procrastination. When your 401(k) contribution is automatically deducted every time you are paid, questions like "should I or shouldn't I invest" disappear. In essence, you are eliminating your emotions from your investing. Furthermore, this feature also gives you the benefit of dollar cost averaging—that is, investing the same amount of money at regular intervals, which averages the prices you pay for your investments so that you substantially reduce the chance of buying all your securities at high prices. That enforced regular investing discipline will really pay off when you are ready to retire.

Your plan is portable: Once you are 100% *vested* (that is, once you have the rights to all of the money) in your 401(k) plan, that money is yours to do with as you please. If you leave your job, you can transfer your 401(k) plan funds to a traditional IRA; you will enjoy the same tax-deferred growth in earnings with an IRA as you did with your 401(k) plan. However, be very, very careful when moving your money. Unless all of the transfer paperwork is done correctly, the IRS will consider your entire 401(k) plan taxable as ordinary income in the year it was transferred!

401(k) Drawbacks

Illiquidity: One primary drawback to a 401(k) plan is that you do not have immediate access to your money. These restrictions are greater than a traditional IRA or a Roth IRA plan, so if the fact that your 401(k) locks your money up bothers you in an extreme way, consider not investing or investing a smaller amount.

Limited investment choices: A 401(k) plan will typically limit you in your choice of investment selections, although many 401(k) plans are increasing the number of investment choices offered to employees.

401(k) Plans Make Sense for Most People

All things considered, most 401(k) plans are terrific retirement savings plan for employees. Each employer's plan varies to some degree, but for most people this plan is an excellent way to build a financial foundation for their desired retirement lifestyle.

Choosing the Best Retirement Plan(s) for You

As you can see, there are a number of different retirement savings plans. Which is the appropriate one for you will depend on your particular circumstances. If you are an employee, you will be faced with a different set of retirement savings options from those the self-employed will consider. Regardless of whether you are an employee or owner of a company, if you can qualify for a tax-free Roth IRA, make your full contribution. At this time, it is the only retirement plan that the IRS cannot levy taxes on and the only purely tax-free retirement plan available. Do not ignore your other retirement plan choices, but look first at the Roth IRA.

—*Annuities: Misunderstood Investment*—

If you asked me what the most widely held and misunderstood investment is, my immediate response would be *annuities!* Annuity sales in the United States have skyrocketed in recent years, and this trend is expected to continue well into the 21st century. The problem is that many people who purchase annuities simply don't understand what they are buying. The advertisements for annuities are partially to blame. Some of these ads border on the ridiculous. For instance, one ad will claim that investing in annuities will result in financial catastrophe or that it is a "ticking time bomb" waiting to explode on your heirs. Another equally convincing ad will assure you that annuities are a fantastic investment you can't live without. Which should you believe? The reality in this case falls somewhere in the middle. Depending upon your circumstances and your financial goals and profile, annuities may or may not be appropriate for you. Probably more so than with any other investment, adequate education is paramount. I strongly recommend enlisting the assistance of a nowledgeable, unbiased advisor specializing in annuities, preferably one with the Certified Annuity Advisor professional designation.

What Is an Annuity?

An annuity is an investment you make in contract form with an insurance company. Earnings growth inside the annuity is on a tax-deferred basis—meaning that you pay no tax on interest, dividends, or capital gains until you withdraw money from your annuity contract. When you do withdraw money from your annuity, earnings on the withdrawals are taxed as ordinary income and not as capital gain.

Advantages of Annuities

All else being equal, thanks to tax-deferral, you can accumulate more money over a shorter period of time and, consequently, earn a greater long-term return on your investment with annuities.

The graph on page 140 shows what a major difference a tax-deferred advantage can make. This illustration assumes an initial investment of $100,000 at an 8% annual compounded rate of return in the 30% tax bracket. Over a period of 25 years, the

$100,000 initial investment in a taxable account would grow to $390,479. In a tax-deferred annuity that same $100,000 would have grown to $684,848.

In addition to deferring taxes, annuities allow you to control when you will pay the tax on any built-up gains in your contract. Unlike IRAs, annuities do not dictate minimum distribution rules on when you must begin withdrawing money. Therefore, you can delay taxation on your annuity till a time that is most favorable for you.

Probate: Your beneficiaries will have the accumulated value of your annuity available to them at your death and, in addition, may avoid the expense, delays, and publicity of probate.

Liquidity: Most tax-deferred annuities allow you to withdraw a portion of your annuity value (usually 10% to 15%) penalty-free either immediately or after the first policy anniversary. Furthermore, many annuity contracts allow for penalty-free withdrawal of your entire annuity in the case of your confinement to a nursing home, diagnosis with a terminal illness, or, in some cases, even unemployment.

Guaranteed lifetime income: When you *annuitize* your annuity—that is, when you begin to receive income payments (purchasing an immediate annuity achieves the same result), you can establish a guaranteed lifetime income stream that you cannot outlive.

Annuitizing your annuity provides you with the additional advantage of receiving a portion of your income tax-free. Part of your monthly income is a tax-free return of your initial investment. (This assumes that your annuity is not inside your IRA; in that case 100% of you annuity income is taxable.)

Asset protection: In many states, assets held in annuities and life insurance policies are protected from creditors. People with professional practices—such as doctors, lawyers, CPAs, and financial advisors—are prime targets for lawsuits. Annuities may provide an additional layer of asset protection in the event of a malpractice lawsuit. Be sure to check the legal statutes in your state.

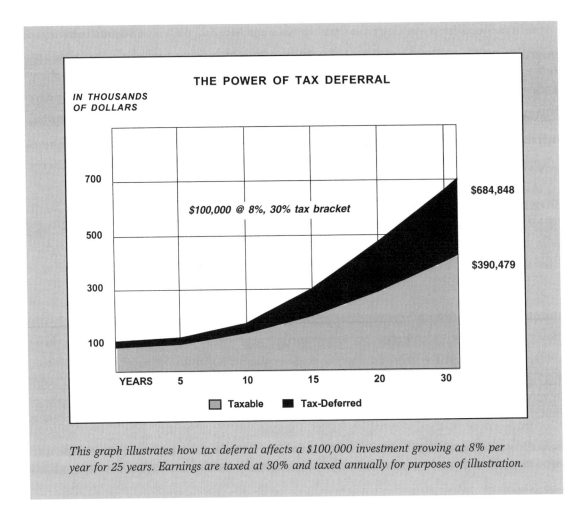

This graph illustrates how tax deferral affects a $100,000 investment growing at 8% per year for 25 years. Earnings are taxed at 30% and taxed annually for purposes of illustration.

Guaranteed death benefit: The vast majority of annuities provide investors with the assurance that, at the death of the annuity owner, the beneficiary will receive no less than the original investment, less any withdrawals. In addition, many annuities offer certain "living benefits," which can be in the form of guaranteed minimum rates of return.

Types of Annuities

Because investors have different goals, risk tolerances, and expectations for performance, the issuers of annuities offer investors a variety of annuities to choose from. There are essentially four different types of annuities.

Immediate Annuity

An immediate annuity does just what its name implies—it pays you an immediate income. Your income is guaranteed for the life of the contract and is paid out partially as a tax-free return of principal. There are two types of immediate annuities:

- The *traditional immediate annuity*, whereby you "trade" your assets for a guaranteed income from the insurance company

- The *variable immediate annuity*, which pays you a varying amount of income that fluctuates according to the investment selections you choose inside your variable immediate annuity. The primary advantage of this annuity is the potential for additional income and inflation protection—assuming that the investment sub-accounts perform well.

Fixed Annuity

Fixed annuities are fully guaranteed in both principal and interest for the life of the contract. Some fixed annuities pay a fixed rate for the contract term, whereas other fixed-rate annuities have a rate that is fixed only for a certain period of time and then is adjusted annually or semi-annually. Be cautious of these adjustable-rate forms of the fixed annuity. I have seen many annuities that started out at 8% or 9% and are now in the 3% to 4% range. Also, be sure to examine carefully fixed-rate annuities that offer a "bonus" feature. While some bonus plans can make sense in your portfolio, with other bonus plans you may ultimately be left with a very low rate of return (under 4%) for years.

If safety of principal, a need for income, and a guaranteed rate of return are your primary concerns, a fixed annuity may serve your purposes.

Variable Annuities

A variable annuity allows the investor to choose from a wide range of investment options called *sub-accounts*. Most variable annuities offer a selection of stock, bond, and money market sub-accounts. The easiest way to think of a variable annuity is simply as a collection of tax-deferred mutual funds (referred to as investment sub-accounts when inside an annuity). As with mutual funds, you can utilize a diversification or asset allocation strategy and choose the investment sub-accounts that are best suited to your goals and time horizon.

Variable annuities are best suited to investors who want the advantages of both tax deferral and mutual-fund-like investment sub-accounts. Another major advantage of a variable annuity over mutual funds is that your beneficiaries are guaranteed to receive at least the original investment at the owner's death. This can be a very compelling feature, particularly for those whose goals include leaving a legacy for their heirs. In addition, most variable annuities today offer "living benefit" guarantees that help protect and/or provide guaranteed growth during your lifetime. Think of these guarantees as *portfolio insurance,* much like homeowner's insurance.

Equity Index Annuities

Equity index annuities may be most appropriate for investors who wish to earn rates of return above those of CDs or money market accounts but are not entirely comfortable with direct exposure to the stock market.

Equity index annuities are actually a form of fixed annuities and have similar safety features of a fixed annuity. Your initial investment is always guaranteed; and as one of the investment choices, you are typically offered a fixed rate option, usually in the 3%–5% range. In addition to the guarantees, equity index annuities provide exposure to the stock market by way of one or more stock market indexes.

One major disadvantage associated with some equity index annuities is that they participate in only one index, the S&P 500. A much better option may be a *multi-index annuity* approach, which provides you with the choice of participating in several indexes. Several equity index annuity providers allow you to choose among the Dow Jones Industrial Average (DJIA), NASDAQ, NASDAQ100, and Russell 2000 (small stock index), as well as the S&P 500. This approach gives you greater portfolio diversification along with the potential for superior returns while providing the same guarantees as a single index annuity.

Annual Reset Provision

Some equity index annuities offer an *annual reset provision.* This provision allows for an "index credit" (account appreciation) to be added to the investor's account on each anniversary of its opening. Once added, it is locked-in and can never be taken away by future market performance.

This locked-in appreciation is added to the initial investment, and that amount becomes the annuity's new *guaranteed floor.* For example, let's say you invest $100,000 in an equity index annuity that gains 10% in the first year. Your new guaranteed floor is now $110,000, and your annuity value can never fall below $110,000. This feature is especially valuable when the stock market experiences a severe downturn. While mutual fund owners must wait for the stock market to recover from a severe correction before experiencing any gains, equity index annuity contract owners with annual reset provisions have their gains locked-in, so their annuities cannot decrease in value.

Equity index annuities attempt to provide investors with the best of both worlds: the safety of a fixed annuity with stock market participation and its potential for greater investment returns.

1035 Exchange

If for some reason you are dissatisfied with your annuity, the IRS has a provision called the *1035 exchange* that allows you to transfer your existing annuity to another annuity at a different insurance company without incurring any tax. However, before you do this, check for any existing surrender charges you might be incurring. Some annuity providers offer up-front bonuses designed to encourage you to move your money by offsetting surrender charges with the up-front bonus.

Disadvantages of Annuities

While annuities offer many advantages, there are also some significant disadvantages to consider before you invest.

Taxed as Ordinary Income

While earnings in your annuity are tax-deferred, when you do withdraw money from your annuity, the money you take out is taxed as regular income instead of at the lower capital gains tax rate in taxable accounts like stocks or mutual funds. However, only contract earnings are taxed, unlike in a traditional IRA, in which 100% of all withdrawals (principle and earnings) are taxed as ordinary income.

Illiquidity

Most annuities do not give you immediate access to your entire account without charging a surrender penalty. You can typically get 10%–15% of your annuity's value per year penalty-free until the surrender period expires. However, exceptions are allowed by many annuity issuers for terminal illnesses, nursing home confinement, and financial hardship.

Fees and Expenses

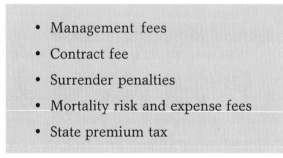

- Management fees
- Contract fee
- Surrender penalties
- Mortality risk and expense fees
- State premium tax

Variable annuities tend to be the most expensive form of annuities when it comes to cost. Remember that, as with most things in life, with investing nothing comes free. Below is a list of fees and expenses associated with variable annuities. Make sure these fees are explained to you in detail before you invest in any annuity.

Early Withdrawal Penalty

If you withdraw funds before you reach age 59½, the IRS will subject you to a 10% early withdrawal penalty.

The Eight Biggest Annuity Mistakes

Many investors make very serious annuity mistakes that cost them, as well as their heirs, a great deal of unnecessary time, money, and aggravation. Here are the eight biggest annuity mistakes and some techniques designed to avoid them.

Mistake #1: Not Fully Understanding the "Parties to the Contract"

If you currently own one or more annuities, I'm sure you remember that filling out the paperwork was somewhat involved. There is a good and valid reason for this. How you fill out your paperwork in terms of designating the appropriate parties or entities (such as a living trust) for your annuity is crucial. These designations will have a major impact on who controls your annuity, who enjoys the tax benefits, who is ultimately entitled to receive the income, and who will receive the annuity proceeds at your death. If you do not currently own an annuity, I am glad you are reading about this mistake before signing your name on the dotted line. It is far too common to see annuity owners who discovered too late that the paperwork was never filled out properly and may not have reflected their true desires. It is of critical importance that you clearly understand the parties involved in your annuity, your role in the annuity, and how setting up your annuity properly can avoid major income tax, estate tax, and estate planning problems down the road.

There are four parties to tax-deferred annuities: the insurance company, the owner, the annuitant, and the beneficiary.

The Insurance Company: By law, annuities must be issued by a life insurance company. It is vitally important that you obtain detailed information about the insurance company with whom you are investing all or part of your nest egg. The first thing you will want to know about the insurance company is how it scores with the respected insurance rating agencies. These ratings are based on the insurance company's ability to meet policyholder obligations, its financial strength, and its operating performance. These rating agencies are the *Consumer Reports* of the insurance industry. At a minimum, be sure to obtain the A. M. Best, Standard & Poors, and Weiss and Fitch ratings on your insurer. For example, the top rating issued by A. M. Best is A + +; however, an A + rating is also considered "superior."

The second key piece of information to uncover about the insurance company is what types of investments it makes with its assets. High-quality corporate bonds, U.S. government bonds, U.S. governmental agency bonds, and other conservative investments are good signs of a stable investment portfolio.

The Owner: The contract owner is the person entitled to exercise all rights under the contract, otherwise known as "incidents of ownership." The owner has the right to the cash surrender value in the contract. The owner can also name the beneficiary and change the designated beneficiary as he or she desires. The owner also receives all tax benefits of the annuity during the accumulation phase (the period before annuity payments begin). The owner of the annuity is frequently the *annuitant* as well. The owner may be an individual or a trust; if you do have a trust, be sure you understand the pros and cons of both choices before making your decision as to whether your trust should be the annuity owner.

A major and often overlooked option when setting up the ownership of an annuity is whether to name a *co-owner.* One advantage of co-ownership is that, in the event of the death of one of the owners, the surviving owner may elect to continue the contract with no tax consequences. However, be aware that with most annuity issuers, in order to avoid the tax consequences at death *the co-owner must be your spouse!* If you are married, I would not recommend naming anyone other than your spouse as co-owner unless you have written consent from your spouse. As always, each insurance company has its own policies regarding ownership, and you should rely on the prospectus and/or your financial advisor (who should be intimately acquainted with the prospectus) to be sure that you are complying with the policies and procedures of the insurance company.

The Annuitant: The annuitant is any natural person (or persons) whose life is used to determine the terms of the annuity payments. The annuitant is entitled to receive all annuity payments under the policy during the *income phase* (more commonly referred to as annuitization or an immediate annuity). A contract may have more than one annuitant (also known as a co-annuitant).

The Beneficiary: The beneficiary is the person(s) or entity (such as a trust) whom the contract designates to receive the death benefit proceeds of the annuity. In many annuity contracts, if the spouse is named as sole beneficiary, that spouse may elect to continue the contract with no taxes due. Also, you may name more than one primary beneficiary in your contract, as well as multiple contingent beneficiaries. Be sure to check with your insurance company to be sure that their policies allow for this provision. As with the annuitant and ownership designations of your annuity, I highly recommend that, if for some reason (which is unusual) you name anyone other than your spouse as the primary beneficiary, be sure that your spouse agrees to this in writing.

ANNUITANT VS. OWNER-DRIVEN CONTRACTS

Another major pitfall experienced by the parties to an annuity is the rarely discussed "Annuitant Driven" contract versus the "Owner Driven" contract provision. I am shocked at how few annuity owners and annuitants understand this concept and appreciate its significance (and potentially negative consequences).

All annuity contracts are either owner-driven or annuitant-driven. With an owner-driven contract, the owner's death will trigger the death benefit; conversely, in an annuitant-driven contract the annuitant's death triggers the death benefit. This has tremendous significance and implications, particularly in cases where the owner and the annuitant are not the same person. For instance, let's say that you are the owner of an annuity that you obtained either through a divorce or a death. If the annuity contract is an annuitant-driven contract and you are the owner but not the annuitant, upon the death of the annuitant, 100% of your annuities value will be paid to the designated beneficiary on the contract. In other words, while you are alive, 100% of your annuities value could be taken away from you at the death of the annuitant, whoever that may be. How's that for a jaw dropping surprise? Don't let it happen to you!

Mistake #2: Not Taking Advantage of the Guarantees Available

The choices available to annuity consumers have never been greater or more misunderstood, but these choices are considerable compared to what existed just a few years ago. Traditionally, annuities came with a standard "death benefit guarantee," but recently all that has changed with additional guaranteed options now available. Before you can make appropriate choices, it is important to become educated on the subject. Four major types of annuity guarantees are offered:

1. ***Standard Death-Benefit Guarantee:*** This is the traditional guarantee most commonly associated with annuities. It is also the most frequently mentioned annuity guarantee. The standard death-benefit guarantee usually says something such as this: "The death benefit shall be the greater of the contract value or the sum of all purchase payments made, less any withdrawals."

    There is a great deal of variance from one company to the next regarding death-benefit provisions. It is vitally important that you examine the standard death-benefit provisions from your annuity provider.

2. ***Annual Step-Up Guarantee:*** This guarantee is an annual "step-up" minimum death benefit, which locks in investment gains on your contract anniversary with the highest value. In other words, each anniversary year starting with your annuity contract's inception date, the insurance company will look to see if your account value is higher than your last anniversary date. If the value is higher, your contract's minimum guaranteed death benefit will "step up" to that new value, and it will never go below this amount. Your annuity now has a new "floor" which it can never fall below. Equity Index Annuities have been traditionally associated with this type of guarantee (also known as the annual reset provision); however, some variable annuity providers now offer it, often at an additional cost. As always, each issuer's guarantee will vary, so be sure to check the company's prospectus.

3. *Guaranteed Earnings Benefit:* This is a nice estate-planning technique you can use to help offset taxes, pay expenses, and provide your spouse with the ability to continue building wealth, as well as pass on more wealth to your children. It is particularly helpful in cases where the owner of the annuity policy is in poor health and cannot get favorable underwriting on estate-planning life insurance. While this benefit is not technically life insurance, it can be used as an effective replacement with no medical underwriting required or minimum health requirements whatsoever. Typically, most guaranteed earnings benefits provide for an additional percentage of contract earnings to be paid to your heirs at your death. Here's a hypothetical example of how this might work:

> Initial investment $150,000
>
> Contract value appreciation $100,000
>
> Contract value at owner's death $250,000
>
> * Guaranteed Earnings Benefit .... **$40,000** (40% of $100,000)
>
> Total death benefit at owner's death ... $290,000

In this case, the annuity provider will pay you 40% of the contract value's appreciation as your guaranteed earnings benefit. Therefore, the total guaranteed earnings benefit is $40,000, which is 40% of the $100,000 contract value appreciation. Guaranteed earnings benefits will vary from company to company, but if you are medically uninsurable, this feature may be worthy of your consideration.

4. *Guaranteed Minimum Retirement Income:* This is a "living benefit," one which you may benefit from while alive. This benefit allows you to enjoy the best of both worlds: market gains when they occur and a "safety net" for your retirement income if the market falters.

Here's how this type of guarantee might work for you:

- If stock market falls, you are assured that a guaranteed income base (up to 7% compounded annually, depending upon the issuer) can provide guaranteed lifetime payments.

- If the market performs well, a "step-up" feature, similar to the annual step-up guarantee I discussed previously, locks in the highest contract anniversary value.

The guaranteed retirement income benefit allows you the luxury of either enjoying the gains of the markets or exercising your minimum interest rate guarantee, whichever choice is most advantageous to you. As always, check the prospectus, as all guarantees of this type will vary from issuer to issuer.

With the unpredictability of global economics and the continued likelihood of terrorism, I strongly suggest that you look seriously at all of the annuity guarantees available as a way to protect your portfolio from adverse events and market volatility.

Tax-Free 1035 Exchange*: This is a tax-free transfer of your annuity or IRA annuity from one company to another, which the IRS allows. The decision to move your annuity to another company should be based on a thorough understanding of your needs, the choices available, and the benefits of such a move.

Mistake #3: Falling Victim to the "Fixed" Rate Annuity Illusion

Many annuity investors purchase what are commonly referred to as "guaranteed* fixed-rate annuities." Not all fixed-rate annuities are created equal, and the "fixed rates" of some annuities are really just temporarily fixed. A more accurate definition of these so-called "fixed" annuities would be "adjustable rate" annuities.

The investor in many cases assumes that the annuity rate is "guaranteed" for the life of the annuity—and many times couldn't be more wrong! What was purchased is an annuity "fixed" for only a certain period of time (say six months or one year) which then adjusts annually or semi-annually after that. Buyer beware!

---

* This guarantee is based on the claims-paying ability of the issuer.

I have seen many annuities that started out at 8%–9% and have gone down to 3%. Also, be aware of fixed rate annuities with a "bonus" feature. While there are some "bonus" plans that can make sense, you could get stuck with a very low return (possibly 3%–5%) for years. Interestingly, I have yet to see one of these "fixed/adjustable" rate annuities where the rate actually goes up over a long period of time! Also, remember to factor in the rate of inflation. With inflation running between 2% and 3%, every additional percent of interest on your annuity is crucial to your bottom line. For instance, on a $100,000 annuity just by earning an additional 2% per year, you could earn an extra $10,408 in just five years ($100,000 @ 2% interest for 5 years = $10,408)!

So what's an annuity investor to do? Using the 1035 exchange or "tax-free exchange," you can move your existing annuity to a new annuity with better rates and terms—and do it tax-free! Note that your existing annuity may assess surrender charges (a competent financial advisor can help you look into that). The bottom line is that, if you want a true "fixed-rate" annuity, there are many good quality insurance companies that offer them. Weigh your options carefully when exchanging your annuity for a new one. A tax-free exchange may or may not be to your best advantage.

Mistake #4: Incomplete Information on Equity Index Annuities

Equity index annuities can be a smart choice for some investors; however, many investors often purchase them without a complete knowledge of the advantages and disadvantages or of the different types of equity index annuities available.

Many equity index annuities have the following features in common:

- The performance is dictated by a percentage of the returns of the S&P 500 index. The S&P 500 index is an unmanaged stock market index of the 500 largest companies in the United States.

- Your principal may be guaranteed at death (payable to your beneficiary) by the insurance company who issued the annuity.

An equity index annuity may be most appropriate for investors who wish to participate in the stock market but are not entirely comfortable with the volatility of direct stock exposure (such as stocks or stock mutual funds). Also, if you seek potential returns greater than those in fixed-income investments such as CDs or high-quality bonds, equity index annuities may be the next logical step for you. If you have a fixed-rate annuity that has suffered a serious interest rate drop (say from 9% to 3%), an equity index annuity could be an attractive alternative.

Due to the way equity index annuities are designed—more as a souped-up fixed annuity than a variable annuity—you should not expect the same type of upside potential as you might get with equities or a variable annuity. Another disadvantage associated with some equity index annuities is that you participate in the performance of only one index—the S&P 500 Index. A much better option is a multi-index annuity that gives you the choice of participation in several indexes, such as the Dow Jones Industrial Average, NASDAQ 100, Russell 2000 (small stock index) as well as the S&P 500. This can be a much more desirable approach giving you greater portfolio diversification and the potential for greater returns while providing guarantees similar to those of a single index annuity.

As part of your equity index annuity evaluation, I highly recommend that you consider as an alternative the new breed of "guaranteed" variable annuities now available. Also, realize that some financial advisors that may be promoting equity index annuities (as this requires that they have only an insurance license) and may not be discussing variable annuities (which would require insurance and NASD securities license) because they do not have the appropriate licenses to legally discuss them with you. Choose a financial advisor who will explain all of your alternatives to you without limitations.

Mistake #5: Not Annuitizing When Most Advantageous

There seems to be no end to misconceptions and misinformation about annuities. Nowhere is this more prevalent than on the subject of *annuitization,* the process whereby you begin to receive income payments from your annuity provider. One of the questions most frequently asked by annuity owners goes something like this: "I once heard that I should never annuitize my annuities; is this true?" Curiously, many annuity owners who have pondered this question can't remember where they heard the "never annuitize" commandment. Wherever it was, the statement "never annuitize" is simply incorrect. Annuitizing isn't for everyone, but it is one of a host of annuity benefits that should be understood and evaluated by every annuity investor.

Let's discuss some annuitization basics to get an understanding of the fundamentals. First, realize that the words *annuitize, annuitization,* and *immediate annuity* mean the same thing; they all refer to taking income from your annuity according to an agreement between you and the insurance company.

There are many different ways you can take the income; without a complete examination of each one, I will recommend that you look carefully at every alternative. Some of the benefits of annuitizing are as follows:

- Part of your income is a tax-free return of principal that can lower your income taxes and Social Security income taxes.

- You can set up your pay-out so that you are guaranteed to receive at least your entire investment back in the form of income payments.

- If you annuitize correctly, after your death your heirs can continue to receive payments that are partially tax-free.

- You can get inflation protection with a special type of "immediate annuity."

- You can create a stream of income that you can never outlive.

The decision to annuitize or to invest in an immediate annuity is one that must be made with a clear understanding of the reasoning behind such a decision and of the benefits that it will bring to you and your heirs. Also, never assume that the insurance company you currently have your annuity with can offer you the best annuitization. This is a very common mistake.

The decision to annuitize may have a profound impact on your financial future and that of your heirs. Because of this, I strongly urge you to educate yourself in this area or work closely with a financial advisor who has extensive annuity experience. If you own an annuity or plan to own one, this decision could be the most significant one you make in your lifetime. And if you think the IRS isn't just waiting for you to make a big annuity mistake, think again.

Mistake #6: Failure to Create Maximum Wealth for Heirs

If you could only pick one mistake to avoid when planning your annuity, pick this one, because it's a whopper. Many, many annuity owners are guilty of simply investing in an annuity without realizing that, if it is not handled properly, the IRS is just waiting with open arms to tax you and your beneficiaries to the maximum.

The first thing to remember is that what the IRS gives you, the IRS would simply love to take away. In the case of your annuity, the IRS is allowing your dividends, interest, and earnings to grow tax-deferred, not tax-free. The good news is that you are using profits from your annuity that otherwise would have been paid to the IRS on April 15th in the form of income taxes to help compound the growth of your annuity. However, the IRS is just waiting patiently to get what it can from you.

Here is a hypothetical illustration of how you can maximize the wealth for your heirs: Helen, an annuity owner, makes an initial annuity investment of $100,000 at age 60; and ten years later her annuity is now worth $200,000. No tax has been paid to the IRS, and Helen is quite pleased with her investment choice of ten years earlier. However, at Helen's death her beneficiaries can be in for a nasty surprise. In this case, with no further planning, here is what would happen at Helen's death:

Total Annuity	$200,000
Federal Income Taxes	– 28,000 (assumes 28% tax bracket)
To heirs after taxes	$172,000

Helen's beneficiaries would pay taxes on the $100,000 taxable gain in the $200,000 annuity, which amounts to $28,000 (28% x $100,000).

Rather than sit and wait for the IRS to dictate to her how much money she could leave to her heirs, Helen decides to proactively manage her annuity in order to maximize the inheritance to her heirs. She chooses to leverage her annuity to create substantially more wealth for her heirs. Let's take a look at how Helen did that and how you can do it too.

First, you must look into what, if any, surrender charges may apply to your annuity. Also, if you are under the age of 59½, a 10% tax penalty may apply. Once this has been determined, you now "annuitize" your annuity. This simply means that you trade in your annuity for a guaranteed lifetime income (or another period of time that you prefer). If you don't already have an annuity, you can purchase an immediate annuity and essentially accomplish the same thing.

In Helen's case, her guaranteed annuity income with an "installment refund" payout is $1,481 per month* based on her $200,000 premium. With the installment refund option chosen, Helen is guaranteed to receive payments until her death, and her heirs will also be guaranteed to receive any remaining payments. With this extra income, Helen can purchase a universal life insurance policy with herself as the insured and her beneficiaries acting as the owners of that policy. This allows the life insurance death benefit to pass outside of Helen's estate, resulting in $0 of income and estate tax due on the life insurance death benefit proceeds.

---

* For illustration purposes only, your payout will be dependent on a number of factors such as your age, gender, interest rates, insurance company calculations, and other factors.

Let's suppose that Helen is in good health and a nonsmoker, and her $1,481-per-month annuity income pays for a preferred-rate $750,000 life insurance policy.**

Look what a major difference this planning will make for Helen's beneficiaries. If Helen had done nothing with her annuity, her beneficiaries would have received a paltry $172,000 after income taxes. With the annuitization of her annuity and purchase of life insurance with the proceeds, Helen's heirs will receive $750,000 in the form of an income- and estate-tax-free death benefit at Helen's death. This is a very powerful tax planning technique!

Mistake #7: Social Security Income Tax—Less Is Better

In 1993, Congress legislated that up to 85% of Social Security income could be taxed. This is just another form of creative taxation by the IRS. I have discovered over the years that most folks do little if anything to combat the IRS in its efforts to tax Social Security income. One major reason is that, because the IRS makes the tax calculations overly complicated, many investors simply don't know what their tax bill will be until they receive an unpleasant surprise on April 15th.

The IRS taxes your Social Security income based on "threshold income" (the IRS definition for income subject to Social Security Tax). This is income from all sources except tax-deferred annuity income left in the contract to accumulate (reinvested) or the tax-free portion of your immediate annuity payout (annuitized income).

Therefore, by replacing existing investments with an annuity (subject to your financial planning objectives), you could reduce or eliminate the tax on your Social Security income. Tax-free municipal bonds and U.S. Treasury Securities will not reduce or eliminate the tax on your Social Security Income.

By correctly calculating the Social Security tax on your income, you will have a clear picture of how much of an annuity investment it would take to reduce or eliminate

---

** For illustration purposes only, your benefit will be dependent on your age, medical condition, sex, type of insurance, cost of insurance, and other factors.

your Social Security tax. If you can reduce your adjusted gross income below $25,000 for a single taxpayer and below $32,000 for a married-filing-jointly taxpayer, you will entirely eliminate tax on your Social Security income.

Mistake #8: Financial Devastation from Long-term Care

The financial impact of long-term care can be devastating, particularly if it is for a very long period of time. Currently, one year in a nursing home can cost between $30,000 and $100,000. The impact upon surviving spouses can be financially devastating as well. Seventy-five percent of all nursing home residents are women. Two out of every five Americans age 65 and older will likely enter a nursing home, and more than 20% will be there longer than five years. Factor in an aging baby-boomer population totaling 80 million, and the fact that most Americans in general are living longer, and we have something of a national long-term-care crisis on our hands.

Medicare and Medicare Supplements are grossly inadequate and pay for only a very small percentage of long-term-care costs. If you are wealthy enough, you could go the long-term care insurance route. If you are going to buy this type of insurance, I recommend considering an inflation rider to cover the ongoing impact of inflation on the coverage. Long-term care insurance premiums are extremely expensive (easily thousands of dollars a year for age 65+); and if you never need long-term care, your payments are generally not refundable.

Anyone with enough money to pay for long-term-care insurance should also seriously consider the self-insurance route as an alternative. The money you save by not purchasing the insurance can be used to help grow your investment portfolio. Annuitizing (taking income) from an appreciated annuity can be an excellent way to provide for long-term care expenses as well as eliminating the need for nursing home insurance. In addition, if a long-term-care stay never materializes, you can use the income for whatever you like.

The long-term care alternative that is often overlooked is the use of annuities to enable you to qualify for the Medicaid (Medi-Cal in California) Program. Medicaid is a joint federal/state program that pays long-term care expenses for people with limited income and assets. Medicaid rules and regulations are very strict, vary from state to state, and you must comply with them exactly in order to qualify.

As with your other investments, seek out investment information that is unbiased and not based on your financial advisor's realizing additional commissions or profits from the sale of company-owned, proprietary investments (annuities, in this case). It will take you some time to thoroughly investigate whether annuities have a place in your investment portfolio. Even if they don't, the knowledge you gain will help you improve the quality of your long-term investment decisions.

—*Your Ultimate Retirement Lifestyle*—

As you design your ultimate retirement lifestyle, determining which retirement plan(s) best suit your needs becomes a critical decision. The decisions you make today will have a profound impact on the financial component of your future lifestyle and the realization of that lifestyle goal. Choose wisely and the benefits that you will receive could be much greater than you ever imagined possible.

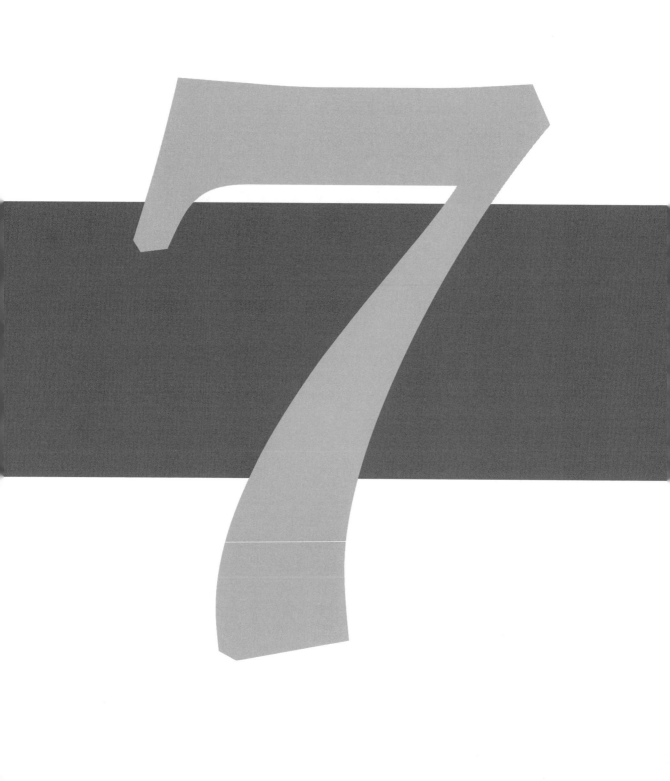

CHAPTER SEVEN

In Search of the Fountain of Youth

In Search of the Fountain of Youth

It's never too late to be the person you want to be.

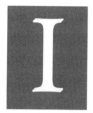n the early 1500s a Spanish explorer named Ponce de Leon journeyed to the New World in search of the legendary "Fountain of Youth." While Ponce de Leon never did find the magical fountain that he was desperately seeking, you can begin your own journey to seek your own personal fountain of youth. In order to keep looking, feeling, and thinking young throughout your life and maintaining your zest for life, you do not need to travel to some exotic faraway place as Ponce de Leon did. Your ability to reverse the effects of aging, achieve your optimal weight, lower your blood pressure, strengthen your immune system, fight cancer, feel great, and live much longer than you ever dreamed possible is well within your reach.

As with any journey, it all begins by taking that first step, even if it's a "baby step." Yours is a journey to better health—to feeling much more alive and excited about life. Let's take the trip together. And because the benefits are much too wonderful to wait another second, let's get started now!

—Balanced Nutrition—
Your Foundation for Good Health

"If we could give every individual the right amount of nourishment and exercise, not too little and not too much, we would have found the safest way to health."
Hippocrates, known as the Father of Modern Medicine, 460–377 B.C.

In order to have a basic understanding of the nutritional habits of most Americans today, it isn't necessary to read some clinical study from a prestigious medical school. The only thing you need to do is go to your local shopping mall and watch as the people go by. You will soon notice how overweight many of the people are. Yes, our fellow Americans. In a nation that takes such pride in education, it is embarrassing how overweight and out of shape most Americans are today. The stark reality is that Americans are slowly killing themselves, and bad diets and poor nutritional habits are two of the main culprits.

Consider these shocking statistics released by the U.S. Department of Health and Human Services ("The Surgeon General's Call to Action to Prevent and Decrease Obesity," 2002):

- Approximately two thirds of United States adults are obese or overweight, as determined by the National Institutes of Health "Body Mass Index," 1998.* This is a jump of 74% in the past 10 years.

- Obesity cost the U.S. economy $117 billion in 2000.

- 13.7% of children aged 6 to 11 and 14% of those aged 12 to 19 were overweight in 1999. The number of overweight children tripled in the previous two decades.

- 300,000 deaths each year in the U.S. are associated with obesity.

- 40% of U.S. adults do not participate in any leisure-time physical activity.

---

* For an explanation of the Body Mass Index, turn to page 225.

According to the American Diabetes Association, over 17 million Americans have diabetes (including an estimated 5.9 million undiagnosed), costing the U.S. $132 billion (up from $98 billion in 1996) in direct medical expenses, lost workdays, restricted activity days, mortality, and permanent disability (*Diabetes Care*, Volume 26, #3, March 2003).

The American Cancer Society predicted the following information on cancer ("American Cancer Society, Cancer Facts and Figures 2003"):

- 1,334,100 new cancer cases to be diagnosed in 2003

- 556,500 Americans expected to die from cancer in 2003— over 1,500 per day

- One-third of the 556,000 cancer deaths in 2003 related to nutrition, obesity, lack of exercise, and other lifestyle factors—all of these deaths avoidable

- 180,000 of the cancer deaths in 2003 resulting from tobacco use

The National Institutes for Health estimates cancer costs at $171.6 billion for 2002. In the United States in 2003, cancer was the #2 killer, accounting for 25% of all deaths and exceeded only by heart disease.

The news on strokes and high blood pressure is also frightening. According to the American Heart Association ("2003 Heart and Stroke Statistical Update"), heart disease is the number one killer of men and women in the United States. Each year approximately one million Americans will have a heart attack, and 500,000 will die. Worldwide, over seven million deaths per year are attributed to heart attacks.

- In the U.S., stroke is the third leading cause of death (only cardiovascular disease and cancer cause more deaths) and is the number one cause of adult disability. Each year 700,000 Americans suffer a stroke and 160,000 die (*WebMD Medical News*, December 2001).

- UCLA Medical Center researchers, led by Dr. Megan C. Leary, report that 11 million Americans suffer "silent strokes" each year. A silent stroke is characterized by tiny spots of dead cells inside the brain but does not cause classic stroke symptoms. When repeated strokes are included, the total goes up to an astounding 22 million silent strokes per year in the U.S. alone (conference of the American Stroke Association, Ft. Lauderdale, Florida, February 9, 2001).

- 50 million Americans have high blood pressure (hypertension), and about 15 million of them don't even know it! High blood pressure is appropriately called the "silent killer" (*Mayo Clinic Health Information,* September 2000).

Americans are simply killing themselves, and much of it has to do with being overweight and in poor physical condition. Of course, factors such as smoking, negative stress, environmental pollution, and lack of exercise contribute to the problem. However, positive health habits and fitness tend to go together. If you are fitness-oriented, you will tend to have a better diet than someone who gets no exercise. Conversely, those who have good nutritional habits tend to be more highly motivated to engage in some form of exercise, such as aerobics or strength-training activities.

As in building the foundation for your home, building your daily nutrition provides the foundation for a long, healthy, and vital life. As in any effort, it is vital to grasp the fundamentals. There is a tremendous amount of misunderstanding regarding what good nutrition is and what it is not. New research has uncovered greater insights as to what is and what is not nutritious. Some whole foods that once were considered bad for you are now viewed as valuable additions to a healthy diet.

It is obvious that the billions of dollars spent on diet drugs, weight loss supplements, and a host of "guaranteed" diets and weight-loss programs have not solved any problems. There is no magical diet pill you can take that will build good health. Instead, proper nutrition must be built upon a solid foundation that will last a lifetime—your lifetime.

The Basics of Good Nutrition

In 1988, the Surgeon General announced that Americans were eating too much fat, particularly saturated fat, and he inaugurated a "war against fat." The government stepped up efforts to encourage Americans to lower their cholesterol and blood pressure. As we shall see, this was easier said than done.

Most Americans embraced the low-fat concept promoted by the government, and the intentions of both the government and the "well-fed" American public were honorable. However, after all these years, Americans have a greater incidence of obesity, high blood pressure, and diabetes than ever before. How could this be? One school of thought is that, in an attempt to eliminate fats from our diets, we have removed many high-quality proteins such as dairy products and meats and replaced them with "fat-free" carbohydrates—often "refined" carbohydrates, such as cookies, snacks, and breads— full of sugar and synthetic ingredients. It's time to get back to the basics of good nutrition. I'm going to help you do this by arming you with the latest research in proper nutrition.

—*The Three Basic Food Groups*—

All foods can be grouped into three basic categories: carbohydrates, fats, and proteins. Let's take a look at all three and I'll show you the role each group plays in your good health and tell you some startling facts research studies have uncovered about them.

Carbohydrates

Carbohydrates are the primary fuel source for your body. Regardless of what you hear on TV infomercials or see in the latest weight loss diet books regarding carbohydrates, they are necessary for good health, and some provide necessary vitamins, minerals, energy, anti-oxidants, and phytochemicals (plant nutrients).

There are two types of carbohydrates: *simple carbohydrates*, such as table sugar, and *complex carbohydrates,* such as fruits, vegetables, potatoes, and pasta. However, an often overlooked problem with carbohydrates is that—regardless of whether you are eating raw sugar, fruits, vegetables, bread or even pure honey—they all are ultimately converted into sugar by your body. This conversion happens at varying rates of absorption.

The second problem with carbohydrates is that, in this era of "low-fat" foods, Americans now eat vast quantities of foods that *appear to be* low in fat, such as fat-free cookies, low-fat potato chips, muffins, etc. The culprits here are refined carbohydrates, the processed foods you see primarily in the bread or snack aisle of your supermarket. Here are some examples of refined carbohydrates:

- Bagels
- Cake
- Chips
- High fructose corn syrup
- Doughnuts
- Honey
- Molasses
- Pie
- White bread
- White flour

Many Americans are addicted to refined carbohydrates. It is crucial that you reduce the amount of these carbohydrates in your diet. They provide little in the way of actual nutrition and, over the long run, can actually be quite dangerous to your health.

INSULIN AND THE GLYCEMIC INDEX

A meal containing any carbohydrate will cause the level of sugar in the blood (blood sugar) to rise to some degree. In response to your elevated blood sugar level, the pancreas secretes insulin, which brings your blood sugar back to normal levels. Depending on how quickly they are absorbed into your bloodstream, different carbohydrates will raise your blood sugar levels by varying degrees. The measure of the absorption rate of carbohydrates is called the *glycemic index.* The greater the glycemic index of the carbohydrate, the greater the rise in blood sugar levels and the more pronounced the rise in insulin levels. Excess insulin is what causes the body to transform carbohydrate calories into fat that becomes stored in the body.

Glycemic means "sugar." The major difference between low-glycemic and high-glycemic carbohydrates is in the fiber and sugar content. More fiber means slower absorption. Therefore, carbohydrates with low sugar and high fiber have the lowest glycemic indexes.

Chronically high insulin and blood sugar levels are hazardous to your health. Health problems associated with high blood sugar levels and elevated insulin levels include:

- Increased free radical cell formation (damage to your body from different kinds of stress) that interacts with cholesterol, which damages arteries and pre-stages blood clots

- Increased LDL ("bad") cholesterol and decreased HDL ("good") cholesterol

- Thicker blood, which is more prone to clotting

- Increased hypertension and heart disease

- Increased chance of developing type 2 diabetes

SOLUTION FOR THE CARBOHYDRATE DILEMMA

By now you may be wondering whether you want to eat any carbohydrates at all. However, don't lose sight of the fact that carbohydrates are necessary for good health. They provide important B vitamins, calcium, and potassium and may protect against heart disease and cancer.

The way to manage carbohydrates is to eat the right types in the right quantities. Stay away from refined carbohydrates like snack foods and baked goods, which are loaded with table sugar and synthetic ingredients including artificial sweeteners and are usually laced with saturated oils. Limit consumption of foods on the high end of the glycemic index—such as candy, doughnuts, white bread, cereals (except for whole grains like as All-Bran), and television snack foods.

The carbohydrates that should make up the bulk of your intake are foods from the low end of the glycemic index. Fruits such as apples, pears, berries, cherries, peaches, melons, oranges, and grapefruits are excellent. Mushrooms and vegetables like avocados, broccoli, eggplant, leafy greens, asparagus, cabbage, and cauliflower are loaded with nutrients, enzymes, and fiber. The tomato, which contains lycopene, beta-carotene, and vitamin C, is appearing in more and more research as a cancer-fighting carbohydrate.

Below I present my recommended list of carbohydrates. Use this list to provide balance and variety in your food selection and to ensure that you are eating carbohydrates with favorable glycemic index ratings. Many of these foods have been shown to be beneficial in preventing heart disease and cancer.

RECOMMENDED CARBOHYDRATES

Fruits	*Vegetables*	*Grains*
Apricots	Asparagus	All-bran cereal
Apples	Brussels sprouts	Barley
Blackberries	Broccoli	Bran, oat
Blueberries	Cabbage	Bran, wheat
Cantaloupe	Celery	Brown rice
Cherries	Eggplant	Buckwheat
Grapefruit	Garlic	Bulgur wheat
Grapes, red	Leafy greens	Couscous
Oranges	Onions	Oatmeal
Peaches	Peppers, red bell	Wheat germ
Plums	Sweet potatoes	Whole-grain bread
Raspberries	Tomatoes	Whole-grain pasta
Strawberries	Spinach	

White potatoes, bananas, corn, carrots, and beets are relatively high on the glycemic index scale. While these foods do offer good nutritional value, they may increase blood sugar levels at a higher rate than my recommended carbohydrates do. Of course, some occasional treats—such as ice cream, real maple syrup, or chocolate—can be good for your emotional well-being if eaten *in moderation* and may even be good for your health.

As a general guideline, I recommend that your carbohydrate consumption be composed of the following: 45% vegetables, 40% fruits, and 15% grains. However, the best way to determine which carbohydrate allocation is right for you is to experiment with your diet. I have been experimenting with carbohydrate combinations for over 20 years and can "feel" which carbohydrate mix is working best for me. Remember, no two people are going to have precisely the same carbohydrate requirements. Use carbohydrates from my recommended list whenever possible.

CHOCOLATE: GOOD FOR YOUR HEALTH?

"All I really need is love, but a little chocolate now and then doesn't hurt."
Lucy Van Pelt in the comic strip "Peanuts," by Charles M. Schulz

A recent study by the University of California at Davis suggests that eating chocolate is actually good for your health. Chocolate contains *flavenoids,* compounds that can help maintain a healthy heart, reduce blood clotting, and maintain good circulation.

The study also found that eating chocolate increased anti-oxidant capacity (cancer protection). Anti-oxidants help reduce damage caused by free radical agents in your body. Free radicals destroy cells in your body and accelerate the aging process. The results of the study support earlier research that cocoa has a similar effect on the blood as low-dose aspirin in reducing blood clotting. However, the study warned against substituting chocolate for aspirin. Of course, most chocolate eaten in this country is loaded with refined sugar, so be moderate in your indulgence.

The bottom line with carbohydrates is to eat the right ones and use carbohydrates as part of a well-balanced nutritious diet. Look for "whole grains" in your breads or crackers, avoid soft drinks filled with sugars, and use alcohol in moderation. If you are going to drink an alcoholic beverage, red wine is best; studies have proven it is good for the heart.

SUPERMARKET SHOPPING PSYCHOLOGY

Food manufacturers spend a great deal of time and money trying to lure you to buy the foods that they make the highest profit from selling. Intensively advertised snack foods such as chips, pretzels, cookies, and muffins are placed strategically on supermarket shelves, often in high-traffic aisles at the eye level of the average American female shopper. Food advertisers, who perform extensive research on consumer buying habits, know that the majority of food shopping dollars are spent by women. In addition, refined snack foods that will appeal to small children are usually placed low on the shelves where children shopping with Mom will readily find them.

You should always check the ingredients of all foods that you buy, but be especially careful when reading the ingredients of those products that are most easily accessible on the supermarket shelves. Also, you may find that the most nutritious foods are on the perimeter (along the walls) and near the refrigerated shelves of the supermarket.

GARLIC: CANCER FIGHTER

Being Italian and growing up with parents who are both wonderful cooks, I have eaten my share of garlic. What I didn't realize for most of that time is what tremendous benefits that marvelous herb was providing in the tomato sauce besides great flavor. Substantial amounts of new research indicate that garlic is a powerful anti-oxidant which substantially lowers the risk of developing breast, stomach, and prostate cancer. In addition, garlic has been shown to lower cholesterol and help prevent heart disease.

Fats

Modern nutritional research is changing much of what we know about fats in our diets. Certain fats in moderation can be a healthy addition to a well-rounded and balanced diet. Let's review the fundamentals of fat.

There are four basic types of fats: saturated, hydrogenated, monounsaturated, and polyunsaturated. *Saturated fats* include butter, coconut and palm oils, fat in meats, and dairy fat. Saturated fats are known to increase blood cholesterol levels and should be eaten sparingly. Many snack foods are very high in saturated fats because of the coconut or palm oils they contain.

Hydrogenated fats are also known as *trans-fatty acids* or synthetic ("fake") fats. This category includes margarine and other foods that are frequently called "partially hydrogenated." These fats are absolutely the worst, and I suggest you remove them totally from your diet because they have been found to create free radical damage, increase cholesterol, and harm your immune system. When faced with a choice between margarine and butter, go—very easy, but go—with the more natural choice: butter.

The two types of unsaturated fats are *monounsaturated* and *polyunsaturated* fats. Foods such as olive oil (choose cold-pressed extra virgin), canola oil, avocados, and sesame seeds are grouped in the monounsaturated and polyunsaturated categories. These fats have been shown to increase HDL ("good") cholesterol and lower the risk of heart disease. Your fat intake should be composed primarily of these two types of unsaturated fats.

WALNUTS AND PEANUTS: HEART-HEALTHY NUTS

New research is now telling us that peanuts (as well as peanut butter) and walnuts are beneficial to your health. Both peanut butter and walnuts have been found to lower bad cholesterol and reduce heart disease risk.

In a recent study by the University of California at Davis published in the July 2000 issue of the *American Journal of Clinical Nutrition,* eating walnuts lowered cholesterol among both healthy men and women as well as those with elevated cholesterol.

The U.S. Department of Agriculture (USDA) just finished a thorough test of of peanut butter, which at one time was thought to be laced with synthetic trans-fatty acids. Researchers tested 11 "name brands" and couldn't find detectable amounts of trans-fatty acids in any of them. Researchers at Penn State University found that moderate-fat diets, including peanuts and peanut butter eaten daily, actually lowered blood cholesterol levels and was more effective than a low-fat diet in maintaining levels of HDL ("good") cholesterol and decreasing trigyceride levels (*Journal of Agriculture and Food Chemistry,* Vol. 49, 5:2349–51).

According to the Peanut Institute (as reported on the Web site peanut-institute.org in December 2001), Americans eat a whopping 1.2 billion pounds of peanut butter annually. Somehow, I think we knew all along that peanut butter wasn't only great tasting but was good for our health as well. As with all foods, use peanut butter in moderation as part of a well balanced diet.

Proteins

The fat-phobic craze that began in the 1980s caused many Americans to reduce their intake of protein under the assumption the saturated fat content of the proteins in such foods as beef and eggs was making people fat. While research has made it clear that too much saturated fat is harmful, it is also becoming obvious that a diet rich in lean meats, fish, poultry, beans (especially soy), and, yes, even the much maligned egg is actually very healthy for us.

Many of today's fad diets now promote proteins as the "miracle" food. Lean protein sources are beneficial to your health, but no food group is necessarily better than another food group, and no one food group can perform miracles. You need to eat from all the food groups in order to be healthy and feel great!

Protein is the substance that helps muscles and bones to grow and repairs your body. Protein is also necessary for healthy hair, skin, and organs. Proteins are made up of amino acids, of which there are a total of 22. Of these, 14 are considered *non-essential* because your body produces them. However, eight amino acids are called *essential* because you must provide them through your diet or through supplementation.

Essential Amino Acids	Non-essential Amino Acids
Isoleucine	Alanine
Leucine	Arginine
Lysine	Aspartic Acid

(Essential Amino Acids)	(Non-essential Amino Acids)
Methionine	CarnitineSerine
Phenylalanine	Creatine
Threonine	Cystine
Tryptophan	Glutamic Acid
Valine	Glycine
	Histidine
	Homocysteine
	Proline
	Taurine
	Tyrosine

Protein in food is of two types. The first is *complete protein;* it comes primarily from animal and dairy sources, such as beef, fish, eggs, milk, and chicken. Complete proteins contain all the essential amino acids necessary to build and maintain muscles, bones, and body tissue. The second type—*incomplete protein*—comes from plants and legumes, such as vegetables, seeds, grains, and nuts. Incomplete proteins must be combined with other protein foods for building and maintaining the body.

In 1993, the Food and Drug Administration (FDA) adopted a new method for calculating the *percent of daily values* (usually shown as "% DV") to be printed on food labels. This is called the *protein digestibility-corrected amino acid score* (PDCAAS) and is basically a measure of the protein content and protein digestibility of foods.

The highest PDCAAS is 1.0. Here are some PDCAAS values for some different food proteins:

PDCAAS for Food Proteins

Food Protein	PDCAAS
Soy protein	1.00
Milk protein	1.00
Egg whites	1.00
Beef protein	0.92
Kidney beans (canned)	0.68

As you can see, soy protein, milk protein, and egg whites have the highest possible protein quality.

SEAFOOD AND THE OMEGA-3 FATTY ACIDS

Omega-3 fatty acids are highly polyunsaturated fats. Including them in your diet can

- Decrease sudden cardiac arrest by up to 50%
- Lower the risk of heart disease
- Prevent blood clots
- Support the immune system

The primary reason for the health benefits of omega-3 fatty acids lies in the *eicosapentaenoic acids* (EPA) they contain. The best food sources for omega-3 and EPA is seafood, particularly the cold-water varieties. Below are some protein sources that are highly nutritious as well as being low in saturated fat and cholesterol.

Recommended Seafood Containing Omega-3 Fatty Acids

Bluefish	King Crab	Sardines
Cod	Mackerel	Shrimp
Herring	Salmon (wild)	Tuna

Of course, seafood that is rich in omega-3 fatty acids also has the added benefit of being a great source of protein, low in saturated fats and full of additional vitamins and minerals. Salmon is a great source for vitamin B-12, and sardines are high in calcium and iron.

Seafood is one of the best protein sources you can eat. (Note that eating raw clams, oysters, or mussels can cause serious health risks such as hepatitis.) However, since protein is such a vital part of your nutritional program, it's important to eat a variety of different protein sources. Find protein foods that you enjoy and that taste good to you. Below are some protein sources that are highly nutritious as well as being low in saturated fat and cholesterol.

RECOMMENDED PROTEINS

Lean beef and venison: Having lived a life oriented towards fitness and nutrition, I find there is something I get from eating beef that I just don't get from any other food. Besides being very high in protein, beef is an excellent source of Vitamins B-3, B-12, and zinc. The linoleic acid found in beef may actually reduce the risk of cancer. The main thing to remember about beef is to choose very lean cuts in order to reduce the amount of saturated fats. Use beef in moderation.

Venison (wild deer) has substantially less saturated fat than some beef. The reason is that wild deer eat a diet of natural grass. Venison is not so readily available as beef, but many health food stores carry it, and you can buy it on the Internet.

Buffalo (North American bison): It doesn't seem long ago that many people included buffalo and dinosaurs in the same category—extinct. At one time there were an estimated 60,000,000 to 125,000,000 bison in North America; by the late 1800s there were 1,000 to 1,500. Today, buffaloes have made an astonishing comeback. In 2001 they numbered about 350,000, according to the National Buffalo Foundation. There has been a noticeable increase in consumption of buffalo meat during the past decade. One reason for the increased interest is that most bison are not subjected to the drugs, chemicals, and hormones that many animals raised for their meat are. In addition, a 1996 research study conducted by Dr. Martin Marchello of North Dakota State University concluded that bison meat is a highly nutrient-dense food. Bison meat is extremely low in fat and is very high in protein. According to the USDA, bison has 25–30% fewer calories than ordinary beef or pork. The USDA chart below shows how bison meat compares with some other proteins:

NUTRIENT COMPOSITION

Species	Grams of Fat	Calories	Cholesterol
Bison	2.42	143	82
Beef	9.28	211	86
Pork	9.66	212	86
Chicken (skinless)	7.41	190	89

(from the *USDA Handbook* 8-5:8-10:8-13:8-17)

There is little doubt that bison meat is an excellent choice when it comes to lean protein. Its biggest drawback is the cost—it's much more expensive than beef. However, you will be getting good value for your dollar if you buy this great-tasting, highly nutritious, and very lean protein source.

EGGS

Eggs have got to be the most maligned and misunderstood protein food. For quite some time it has been popular either to throw out the egg yolk and use only the white or to purchase some sort of "egg substitute" in an attempt to get all of the good features of the egg (egg whites are virtually pure protein) and dispose of the bad features of the egg, presumably the downtrodden yolk. I must admit that I was caught up in this anti-yolk movement for quite some time.

However, new research has brought enlightenment to the yolk-versus-no-yolk controversy. Recent studies have found that whole eggs eaten daily in moderation actually increase HDL cholesterol, the type that is associated with a reduction in heart disease. Certainly, you should follow the advice of your doctor in all cases, but it is becoming more and more apparent that eggs are generally very beneficial to most people's health. Here are some of those benefits:

- Egg whites are virtually pure protein and are one of the highest-quality proteins, according to the FDA.

- Eggs are low in saturated fat.

- Eggs contain substantial amounts of Vitamins A, D, E, and B-12 as well as thiamine, riboflavin, pantothenic acid, folic acid, and phosphorous.

- Egg yolks contain lutein and zeaxanthin, nutrients that reduce the chances of macular degeneration (which can lead to blindness) and protect against colon cancer.

- Eggs are an inexpensive source of good nutrition.

There is a new and improved class of eggs now in your supermarket's refrigerated section. Sometimes termed "designer eggs," these eggs are produced from hens that are fed all-natural vegetarian diets loaded with "heart healthy" omega-3 fatty acids, vitamin E, anti-oxidants lutein and selenium—all nutrients found to promote good health. In addition, designer eggs are generally lower in saturated fat than regular eggs. Currently, there is talk of an even more advanced egg, reduced in total cholesterol by over 75% and pasteurized to reduce the risk of salmonella (source: Jose Antonio, Ph.D., "Eggcellent!," *Muscle and Fitness,* March 2001).

With all the research that has been done on eggs and all of the new, improved eggs coming to market, there is still one thing I have witnessed personally that has greatly influenced my attitude on eggs. My dad, who is 86 years of age, has regularly eaten whole eggs his entire life and is in excellent health. Of course, genetics and other factors may have something to do with this, but the main point is that, eaten in moderation, eggs can be a very healthy addition to most people's diets.

SOY

According to a 1999 U.S. Food and Drug Administration Talk Paper, "Diets low in saturated fat and cholesterol that include 25 grams of soy protein a day may reduce the risk of heart disease." That's quite a statement, especially coming from the FDA.

Actually, soy is one amazing protein source. It is the only plant that provides complete protein, which puts it on the same high level as egg whites and milk as a protein source. Here are just some of the numerous benefits of soy:

- Raises HDL ("good") cholesterol

- Significantly lowers LDL ("bad") cholesterol levels

- Provides soy isoflavones (plant chemicals), powerful anti-oxidant protectors

- Helps keep blood vessels flexible and open

- Provides phytoestrogens, which can reduce menopausal symptoms

- Increases bone density to prevent osteoporosis.

Soybeans are naturally brimming with nutrients including the B vitamins, iron, calcium, potassium, and magnesium. Soy has also been shown to assist in weight management, causing your body to store less fat (*American Journal of Clinical Nutrition,* December 2002).

You can get the benefits of soy in a number of different and delicious ways. *Soy nuts* are a nutrition-packed snack and can be added to salads. *Tofu,* a soy-based textured vegetable protein (TVP), can be used in the diet in place of cheese, meat, or poultry. *Soymilk* is a tasty, healthy alternative to milk; it can also be mixed with milk to provide the combined benefits of both. Soymilk is often fortified with calcium and vitamin D. I recommend drinking it as a delicious daily habit. *Tempeh* is made from whole, cooked soybeans formed into a cake; it is used as a meat substitute. *Miso* is fermented soybean paste used for seasoning and in soup stock.

Soy Protein Powder: Soy is an excellent protein to use in your protein shake. According to the FDA's protein digestibility ratings, soy protein is the highest-quality protein you can eat. However, soy protein powders vary widely in quality and nutritional value, so look for these features:

- Guarantee by the certified identity preservation program as *non-genetically modified organism* (non-GMO) soybeans. This will assure you of getting natural soybeans with nothing synthetic or unnatural added.
- *No saturated fat through added ingredients*
- Added vitamins and minerals for complete and balanced nutrition
- *No added synthetic sweeteners*
- *First listed ingredient is not a form of sugar* (fructose, glucose, sucrose, etc.)

Also, your soy protein powder should taste good! I have used soy protein powder in my health shakes virtually every day for the past four years. It is one of the best additions I have ever made to my diet.

Your soy protein shake should be delicious and nutritious, and, most of all, it should make you feel stronger and revitalized. You can get soy protein in chocolate, vanilla, strawberry, or other natural flavors. There is a tremendous difference in the quality of soy protein powders, so choose wisely and enjoy!

Soy Protein Bars: You can also get soy protein in a protein snack bar. As with soy powder, make sure the soy has not been genetically modified. Strive to find a soy bar that has a much higher level of protein than of carbohydrates and contains little or no added sugar. Oh yes, make sure it tastes good too!

CHICKEN AND TURKEY

Americans eat almost three times as much chicken today as they did in 1960. According to the American Dietetic Association, three ounces of skinless, baked chicken drumstick has less total fat than beef tenderloin, salmon, or pork chops; and chicken breast contains much less fat than the drumstick.

There is some misunderstanding about when to remove the skin. Actually, as long as you remove the skin before eating, it makes no difference whether you cook the chicken (or turkey) with or without the skin. Chicken and turkey are both high in lean protein and make a fine choice for your protein requirements.

DAIRY

Low-fat cottage cheese, low-fat yogurt, and low-fat or skim milk are excellent sources of quick protein. Low-fat cottage cheeses tend to have less sugar content than low-fat yogurt and milk, so be sure to check the ingredients on the containers carefully. All dairy products are excellent sources of protein, Vitamin A, Vitamin D, and calcium. Many low-fat dairy products available today are enriched with added vitamins and minerals. By the way, fat-free buttermilk makes delicious, low-fat, Sunday morning blueberry pancakes!

LEGUMES

Legumes (beans and peas) are an often overlooked source of protein and dietary fiber. Beans and peas come in many varieties, including lentils, navy beans, kidney beans, black-eyed peas, black beans, chick-peas, fava beans, and French white beans. Beans and peas provide fiber, potassium, protein, folate, vitamin B-6, zinc, iron, and phytochemicals (plant chemicals). They are also very low in fat.

According to a recent study in the November 26, 2001, *Archives of Internal Medicine,* men and women who ate legumes four times a week had a 22% lower risk of coronary heart disease than those who consumed legumes only once weekly. The results are based on data collected from more than 9,600 Americans over a 19-year period.

When was the last time you had some delicious chili with red kidney beans or some Cuban black bean soup? Maybe it's time to rediscover the nutritious and delicious food called legumes!

The Okinawa Centenarian Study

One of the most amazing studies on aging and longevity was begun in 1976 by a group of researchers who ultimately published a book entitled *The Okinawa Program* (Bradley J. Wilcox et al., Crown Publishing Group, 2001). The subjects were the people of Okinawa, a small island off the coast of Japan. The study examined the lifestyles, diets, exercise habits, genetics, and spiritual beliefs of Okinawan centenarians (people aged 100 or older) as well as other Okinawans over 70 years of age. For many years it was believed that Okinawans lived very long and healthy lives; the scientists wanted to discover whether this was true and, if so, why.

The average life expectancy of Okinawans is longer than that of any other population on earth. As I was writing this book, there were 457 centenarians in Okinawa—34.7 for every 100,000 islanders, the highest percentage of centenarians in any population group in the world. The United States equivalent is ten centenarians per 100,000 people ("Life," *USA Today*, January 3, 2002). In addition, the *average* life expectancy on Okinawa is 81.2 years: 86 for women, 78 for men—the highest life expectancy in the world. Okinawans' life expectancy even tops that of the Japanese population as a whole (including Okinawans), which averages 79.9 years (Japan Ministry of Health and Welfare, 1996).

Consider some of the health-related findings of the study:

- Okinawans suffer 80% fewer heart attacks than Americans, and their heart attack survival rate is twice as high.

- Okinawans have 80% less breast and prostate cancer and 50% less ovarian and colon cancer than North Americans.

- Stroke and dementia are rare.

- Okinawans suffer 20% fewer hip fractures than mainland Japanese, who in turn have 40% fewer hip fractures than Americans (P. D. Ross, et al., *American Journal of Epidemiology* 1991: 133: 801–9).

- Estrogen replacement therapy is rare, yet Okinawan women have a much lower incidence of hot flashes and coronary artery disease.

- Okinawans are physiologically younger than Americans and have higher levels of sex hormones, including DHEA, estrogen, and testosterone.

- Okinawan centenarians are generally optimistic, adaptable, self-confident, and easy-going.

The risk of dying from various types of cancer is much less for Okinawans, as shown in the chart below:

CANCER DEATH RATES
(per 100,000 people)

	Breast	Prostate	Ovarian	Colon
Okinawa	6	3	4	8
Japan	11	3	8	16
Sweden	34	10	52	19
U.S.A.	33	7	28	19

So what is the secret of the Okinawans' success? The primary reason does not lie in their genes, although their genetic makeup has been shown to be a contributing factor. Rather, the main factors involved in their longevity are a healthy diet, regular exercise, a balanced low-stress lifestyle, little alcohol or tobacco consumption, an optimistic attitude, and an integrated health-care approach featuring much greater use of natural tonics and supplements than in the West.

Here are some features of the Okinawan diet:

- *Soybeans* (Okinawans love tofu), which are rich in isoflavones (also called phytoestrogens or plant estrogens). Eating soybeans has been shown to decrease the risk of breast and prostate cancer, reduce bone loss, and decrease the risk of coronary artery disease.

- *Fish* such as salmon, tuna and mackerel that are high in omega-3 oils (fatty acids) and have been found to reduce the risk of heart disease

- *Little or no dairy products or proteins high in saturated fats*

- *Unrefined complex carbohydrates* such as whole grains, vegetables, etc.

- *The practice of hara hachi bu*—ceasing to eat when 80% full.

One other finding from the study bears mention. The Okinawans do not ignore or isolate the elderly. Even though many live alone, Okinawans look out for each other. Neighbors check up on each other. People have a sense of community and shared activities.

We can learn a great deal from the Okinawans. Trends in the West suggest that we may finally be waking up to the realization that many of the nutritional, fitness, and lifestyle habits the Okinawans have practiced for a very long time can be beneficial for us as well.

—*Putting It All Together*— ## *Six Steps to Good Nutrition*

Now that you have a good understanding of the basics of proper nutrition and the best foods to choose from each of the three basic food groups, it's time to put together your nutrition program. Here are six important steps to take in planning a low-fat, highly nutritious diet that also tastes good. It's time to follow the "six steps to good nutrition."

Step 1: Eat a balanced diet.

Eat a wide variety of foods from the three main food groups, focusing on the recommended foods in this section. As dull as "eat a balanced diet" may sound, it is undoubtedly the healthiest approach. However, "balanced" definitely does not have to mean boring! It is important to combine proteins and carbohydrates with each meal you eat. Combining foods creates "food synergy"—different foods eaten together working in concert to provide the "whole is greater than the sum of its parts" effect. By eating a wide variety of whole foods, you will give yourself a better chance to achieve positive food synergy.

Step 2: Eat six small meals a day.

Eat six small meals per day instead of the traditional three. Besides not eating at all, the worst possible thing you can do is to starve yourself and then overeat. This throws your body's mechanisms totally out of balance. Eating smaller, more frequent meals will allow your metabolism to work more efficiently and help you maintain your desired weight. I have been using this "smaller meal" system for over ten years and it has worked very well for me. Have more complete meals for breakfast, lunch, and dinner, along with three nutritious snack-type meals throughout the day. When you leave home, just put your meals in a small cooler with a freezer pack and take them with you. Every morning I make a nutritious (and delicious) protein shake; then I simply pour the shake into a pint container, put that and my protein bar into my small cooler, and now I've got two snack meals to take with me. Along with a quart of water I'm ready to go anywhere!

Step 3: Prepare healthy food.

Prepare your meals by grilling, baking, steaming, or using your microwave. Avoid frying or saturating your food in butter or oil while cooking—it's not necessary to take in all that saturated fat. When you must use oil in cooking, use heart-healthy first-pressed extra virgin olive oil in moderation; avoid synthetic hydrogenated cooking oils and fats such as margarine. If you want a less powerful taste, you can get a lighter olive oil made for sautéing, baking, and stir-frying. Canola oil is another good choice. You can even get these oils in spray cans if you like.

Step 4: Drink plenty of water.

Always drink water before, during, and in between meals. Drink eight to ten 8-ounce glasses of water every day to prevent dehydration and assist in proper digestion of food. If you exercise (I hope you do), your need for water will be even greater. Drink at least 12 ounces of water for every hour of exercise. Soda, juice, coffee, and teas containing sugar and/or caffeine contribute to dehydration and should not be used in place of water. You may add an occasional glass of "heart healthy" red wine to your meal, but not as a substitute for water.

Step 5: Enjoy healthy food.

Where does it say that healthy foods don't taste good? Strive to eat foods that are not only good for you but also taste good. This is an extremely important point. Your healthy eating habits will perpetuate themselves, and you will find yourself consuming less junk food, sugary drinks, and refined carbohydrates. The key is to feel like you are not "missing out" or struggling to eat foods you really don't want to eat. Of course, an occasional pizza, slice of chocolate fudge cake, or a decadent ice cream sundae, especially when enjoyed with good company, can actually be beneficial for the soul. As you have seen, new research shows that a very wide variety of foods can be good for us when eaten in moderation. Discover which healthy foods you like the best, and enjoy!

Step 6: Use Nutritional Supplements.

Buy only high quality nutritional supplements with "full-spectrum" vitamins and minerals as well as anti-oxidant protection. Use the knowledge you gain in this book to be a discriminating consumer when it comes to the supplements you put into your body. Nutrition shakes and protein bars make for highly nutritious, delicious, and satisfying snack meals. When choosing your supplements, shakes, and bars, avoid those with excessive amounts of sugar or with any artificial sweeteners and synthetic ingredients.

—The Mediterranean Diet—

I will never forget Sunday dinners as a child. Whether eaten at home with mom, dad, brother and sisters, or with 30 relatives, Sunday dinners were feasts. Actually, it seemed as if we ate all day. I think that's because we did. Interestingly enough, not one of us was noticeably overweight. Perhaps genetics played a part in this, but being Italian, we were eating what is now referred to as the "Mediterranean Diet."

In recent research studies, such as the Italian GISSI–Prevenzione Study, scientists suggest that not only is the Mediterranean Diet good for lowering heart disease risk; it can protect people who have already had a heart attack. One of the keys to the Mediterranean Diet is replacing the saturated fat in butter with monounsaturated fat found in olive oil. In order to enjoy some of the many health benefits of the Mediterranean Diet, follow these simple guidelines:

- Use cold-pressed extra virgin olive oil in place of butter when cooking. Extra virgin olive oils come in different natural "flavors," so choose the ones you like best.

- Eat more vegetables during lunch and dinner. Tomatoes (used in tomato sauce) are rich in lycopene, a much more potent anti-oxidant (cancer fighter) than beta-carotene. Garlic and onions, staples of the Mediterranean diet, have been shown to lower blood pressure and decrease heart disease risk.

- Increase the amounts of fruit in your diet. Melons, grapes, and berries are excellent fruit choices.

- Add some nuts to your diet. Walnuts and peanuts have been found to be beneficial in preventing cardiovascular disease. Sure they're high in calories, so try a small amount if that's a concern. For a special treat, try some pine nuts in your favorite salad.

- For protein, add more fish to your diet, but certainly lean red meat (as in meatballs) and chicken (for example, chicken Marsala) are healthy additions when used in moderation.

- Try an occasional glass of your favorite red wine with dinner. Research studies suggest that the red and purple grapes used to make red wine may help in reducing heart disease risk. Potent anti-oxidants called flavenoids in the grapes seem to be the primary beneficial ingredient. Studies now show that purple grape juice has similar benefits, so you may want to pour a glass for the kids (but watch out for added sugar!).

—Meal Plans—

Here is a sample eating plan I developed that combines healthy foods into a balanced, nutritionally sound diet. Try it for a while and see how you feel!

Weekday Meal Plan

Breakfast

- SCRAMBLED EGGS AND WHOLE WHEAT TOAST:

    Two whole eggs and one egg white, scrambled

    One slice whole-grain bread with low-fat cream cheese and low-sugar fruit spread

- ¼ cantaloupe

- Nutritional supplements
- 8 ounces pure water

Snack #1

- CHOCOLATE NUTRITION SHAKE:

Chocolate protein powder	Cherries (pitted fresh or frozen)
2/3 cup soy milk	One Tbsp. peanut butter
2/3 cup cold water	Ice

Mix together in blender; serve cold. Sprinkle with toasted wheat germ (optional). Invite a friend over, or share with family!

Lunch

- LOW-FAT CHICKEN SALAD:

4-oz. chicken breast	1 Tbsp. raisins
Celery	Fresh ground pepper
2 Tbsp. non-fat yogurt	¼ tsp. curry powder (optional)
1 Tbsp. low-fat mayonnaise	

Combine ingredients, adding chicken last.

- 8 ounces pure water

Snack #2

- High protein nutrition bar
- 8 ounces pure water

Dinner

- BAKED SALMON:

Lightly coat salmon with lemon juice and extra virgin olive oil and bake at 350° for about 30 minutes.

- Baked sweet potato with cinnamon
- Steamed broccoli with fresh ground pepper and fresh lemon
- 8 ounces pure water

Snack #3

- 100% All-Bran cereal with chopped dates, wheat germ, and soy milk

Weekend Meal Plan

Breakfast

- ORANGE-PECAN FRENCH TOAST:

1 cup skim milk or fat-free buttermilk	½ cup orange juice
2 whole eggs + 1 egg white	½ tsp. cinnamon
1 cup oat flour	½ cup finely ground pecans
½ Tbsp. baking powder	½ tsp. vanilla

Combine ingredients and dip two slices of whole-grain bread into batter. Cook on griddle. Top with low-sugar fruit spread, and sprinkle with cinnamon.

- ½ grapefruit
- Turkey bacon
- Nutritional supplements
- 8 ounces water

Snack #1

- STRAWBERRY NUTRITION SHAKE:

Vanilla protein powder	Strawberries (fresh or frozen)
1 cup skim milk	Ice
1 cup cold water	

Blend together, serve cold—sprinkle on toasted wheat germ (optional).

Lunch

- TURKEY BURGER WITH SWISS CHEESE AND ROASTED RED PEPPER:

    ½ lb. fresh ground turkey breast   Low-fat swiss cheese

    ¼ diced onion   Roasted red peppers (jar or fresh)

    Fresh ground black pepper   Multi-grain hamburger buns

    Combine first three ingredients. Cook burgers, melt cheese on top, and finish with roasted pepper. Place in buns and enjoy with a friend!

- 8 ounces pure water

Snack #2

- High protein nutrition bar or low-fat cottage cheese and apple
- 8 ounces pure water

Dinner

- WHOLE-GRAIN OR "LOW-CARB" LINGUINE AND GRILLED TUNA IN OLIVE-MUSHROOM-BASIL SAUCE WITH CAESAR SALAD:

    Chopped fresh garlic   Salt and fresh-ground pepper

    2 Tbsp. capers   Basil

    Extra virgin olive oil   Raisins (optional)

    Chopped fresh mushrooms   Pine nuts

    1 cup red or white wine (based on your preference)   Parsley

    Green (Spanish) and black (Greek) olives, pitted and chopped

    1/3 lb. whole-grain or "low-carb" linguine

    10 oz. tuna steak

Sauté garlic and capers in olive oil (take care not to burn). Add mushrooms and sauté. Add wine and cook together for 1 minute. Stir in remainder of ingredients except for the linguine and tuna. Cook for 20 minutes.

Lightly coat tuna steak with extra virgin olive oil and fresh ground pepper. Grill on a preheated outdoor or indoor grill about two minutes on each side. After grilling, cut the tuna steak into bite-sized pieces and add to the sauce.

Boil the linguine according to the directions on the box. Drain the linguine in a colander. Add the linguine to the grilled tuna and sauce and enjoy!

Try a glass of your favorite red wine with this dish, and dine by candlelight with someone special!

- SALAD WITH CAESAR DRESSING:

Extra virgin olive oil	Basil
Balsamic vinegar (white)	Fresh lemon juice
Grated low-fat Parmesan cheese	Anchovies (optional)
Fresh garlic (chopped)	Fresh ground pepper

Combine ingredients and pour over Romaine lettuce. Sprinkle low-fat blue cheese on top (optional).

- 8 ounces of sparkling water (such as San Pellegrino)

Snack #3

- "NO-GUILT" DECADENT CHOCOLATE FROZEN YOGURT SHAKE:

Chocolate protein powder

Chocolate frozen yogurt (low-sugar)

2/3 cup cold water

Blend together for a special treat. Grate some low-sugar chocolate on top!

More Healthy Recipes

Anthony's Texas-Style Chili

1 lb. extra lean ground sirloin

2 Tbsp. extra virgin olive oil

½ cup red wine

½ cup chopped onion

4 cloves finely chopped garlic

1 large can peeled whole tomatoes

1 small can tomato paste

1 can dark red kidney beans

Salt and fresh ground pepper to taste

1 tsp. chili powder

1 tsp. cumin

1 tsp. hot sauce

¼ cup fresh chopped cilantro

Heat olive oil and sauté onions and garlic (without burning garlic). Stir in ground beef and brown. Add wine and simmer for 1 minute. Add tomato paste and whole tomatoes and stir. Stir in kidney beans and all other ingredients. Simmer for 1 hour and enjoy!

Butternut Squash and Sweet Potato Soup

2 apples, peeled, quartered, and cored

1 large onion peeled and halved

2 large sweet potatoes, peeled and cubed

1 butternut squash, peeled and halved with seeds removed

2 cans low-fat, low-sodium chicken broth

2 Tbsp. organic honey

1 Tbsp. curry

Place apples and vegetables on a shallow pan coated with canola oil cooking spray. Cook at 400° for 40 minutes or until done. Pour honey over ingredients.

When cooked, purée in food processor or blender, adding some of the chicken broth. Add blended ingredients to large pot and add remaining chicken broth, water and curry. Excellent for an autumn or winter day!

Summer Strawberry Soup

⅔ cup low-fat or fat-free buttermilk   3 cups fresh strawberries

⅔ cup low-fat vanilla yogurt   Mint

Puree buttermilk, yogurt, and strawberries in blender. Chill in refrigerator and serve garnished with mint. Invite a friend, there's enough for two!

Healthy Pasta Pesto

Pasta Pesto originated in the port of Genoa, Italy, as a quick, but delicious meal for Italian sailors. This reduced-fat, reduced-carb version makes as a quick, delicious and nutritious meal for you and your family.

4 cups fresh basil   Freshly ground black pepper

2 Tbsp. pine nuts   Pinch of ground red pepper (optional)

Pinch of salt   ½ cup grated low-fat Parmesan cheese

4 peeled garlic cloves   2 Tbsp. grated low-fat Romano cheese

3 Tbsp. premium extra virgin   ¾ pound organic whole-wheat or low-
olive oil   carb pasta

Combine the first seven ingredients in a food processor or blender and blend thoroughly. Scoop mixture into a large bowl. Blend in Parmesan and Romano cheeses.

Cook pasta al dente (firm), according to directions. Drain the pasta in a colander. Add pasta to the pesto sauce and toss well. Serves 4. Enjoy it with a good glass of your favorite wine!

—*Water: Hydrated Equals Healthy*—

Water makes up about 55% of a woman's body weight and about 60% of a man's body weight. Your body relies on water for many functions, including keeping your body from becoming poisoned by its own waste products. Toxins from the food you eat, in addition to environmental pollutants such as auto fumes and pesticides, must be flushed from your body. Every cell in your body relies on water for the efficient delivery of needed nutrients from food and nutritional supplements.

Almost everyone these days is aware that water is good for us, but most do not realize just how critical it is. Many people suffer from some degree of chronic dehydration. This chronic dehydration puts people into vicious cycles of stress, which causes further dehydration, which in turn causes more stress, etc. When we become dehydrated, we may be laying the groundwork for a host of illnesses, such as high blood pressure, high blood cholesterol, back pain, depression, and obesity.

Exercise and Water: Dehydration Prevention

At just a 2% drop in water as a percent of your body weight, your overall athletic performance declines by 10%–20%. Runners and cyclists lose 2%–6% of their total body weight while sweating in hot weather. Most athletes do not consume nearly enough water to stay hydrated during athletic events, and their performance undoubtedly suffers.

While many people are in a constant state of chronic dehydration, the need for water becomes even more pronounced for those who exercise. Dehydration during exercise is simply a result of insufficient fluid intake. Pay special attention to your fluid intake when the weather is hot (especially if the humidity is high) when you are engaged in continuous exercise or marathon events, and when you are taking any type of medications. Warning signs of dehydration include headaches, cramps, fatigue, lack of energy, and dry lips and tongue. If you allow your exercise to progress long enough without sufficient fluid intake, you could end up with heat exhaustion or heat stroke. Symptoms include:

- Dizziness
- Nausea or vomiting
- Elevated heart rate
- High temperature
- Rapid, shallow breathing
- Reduced alertness or unconsciousness

Dehydration, especially during exercise, is a matter I want you to take very seriously. Here are some tips you can use to avoid dehydration, enjoy your workouts in any type of weather conditions, and exercise at your maximum performance levels:

- Be sure to eat a balanced diet during the 24 hours prior to a strenuous workout day or competitive event. This will promote maximum hydration.

- Always drink plenty of water before, during, and after exercise in regular intervals. If you wait until you feel thirsty, it's too late—you're already dehydrated.

- To promote hydration, drink at least a pint of water two hours before exercise

- Limit beverages with caffeine (coffee, tea, soft drinks, and alcohol), and avoid them completely during exercise; these drinks promote dehydration.

- Wear clothing that breathes. Athletic apparel manufacturers today offer amazing, lightweight fabrics that pull perspiration away from the body, where it evaporates. Choose clothing made from these fabrics, instead of cotton, which soaks up sweat.

- According to the American College of Sports Medicine, when you are exercising intensely for more than one hour, your performance is best maintained with drinks containing carbohydrates (fructose, glucose, or sucrose) and electrolytes. Beverages containing a small amount of sodium are also suggested. However, do not overdo it with these types of drinks. Use them only if you have exercised very intensely and lost a great deal of fluids while sweating. Otherwise, stick with water; it's best for you in most cases.

- On extremely hot days, try to exercise in the morning or early evening.

- Avoid jacuzzis, saunas, and steam rooms after exercising.

One thing is very clear and bears repeating: you should be drinking a minimum of 8 to 10 8-oz. glasses of water every day and increase your water intake up to at least 10 to 12 glasses a day when exercising. I don't go anywhere (including air travel) without a refillable quart jug of water. I hope you will take up the habit of drinking plenty of water right now. It's one of the simplest and most effective nutritional habits you can form, and it can help you look and feel your best for a long time to come!

—*Nutritional Supplements*— *Natural Prescription for Health*

The Great Debate

Today, over 100 million Americans—more than 40% of the United States population— use nutritional supplements. In addition, all signs point towards increased use of nutritional supplements around the world.

Even with the explosive growth in the use of nutritional supplements, a great deal of controversy remains as to whether we need to supplement our diets in order to maintain good health or whether supplements are mostly a waste of money. Those who claim that supplementation is largely "money down the drain" argue that we obtain the nutrients we need from food and that supplementation has little positive effect on health. Proponents of supplementation argue that we need to add vitamins and minerals to our diet to guarantee good health. Let's examine the current state of the nutritional supplement debate.

Should You Take Supplements?

There is a growing body of evidence from scientific research that supplementing our diets with nutrients is beneficial to our health. Also, there is steady growth in numbers of those in the medical community, particularly American physicians, who are now seeing convincing research studies in favor of nutritional supplementation. A growing number of medical doctors are now beginning to incorporate this knowledge into their practices. Ninety percent of Americans are expected to die from heart disease or cancer, so more and more physicians are looking for alternative and/or complementary approaches to traditional medicine in order to protect their patients from these deadly diseases. Many of our physicians, in an attempt to provide patients with a more "natural" approach to health care, have begun to integrate "preventative" and "alternative" medicine into their health care practices. Combining conventional medical care with alternative medicine (including supplements) is called "integrative medicine." There are many reasons that our physicians have begun to embrace a more "natural" approach to health care, including recommending nutritional supplements as part of a health-conscious lifestyle.

One of the better reasons I've seen for physicians to recommend supplementation is given an article entitled "Vitamins for Chronic Disease Prevention in Adults,"which appeared in the *Journal of the American Medical Association.* It states, "Most people do not consume an optimal amount of all vitamins by diet alone . . . it appears prudent for all adults to take vitamin supplements. Physicians should make specific efforts to learn about their patients' use of vitamins to ensure that they are taking the vitamins they should . . ." (*JAMA* Vol. 287 No. 23, 6/19/2002).

Diets Lack Proper Nutrition

Americans are simply not getting the necessary nutrients in their diets. A nutritious diet is unquestionably beneficial to good long-term health, yet it is estimated that more than 50% of Americans don't get the FDA's recommended dietary allowance of nutrients. Many Americans simply are not eating a well-rounded, nutritious diet. Most Americans, particularly working Americans, are so strapped for time due to work, commuting, and family obligations that eating healthy, nutritious meals doesn't happen the way it should. With all the pressures of modern-day, 21st-century society this is certainly understandable, but definitely correctable.

More Quantity, Less Quality

Most of the foods we eat today are mass-produced on farms and ranches in America and across the globe. High-tech farming allows for much greater crop yields; unfortunately, it also results in the soil's depletion of vitamins and minerals. Adding pesticides, chemicals, and fertilizers to the soil depletes the nutritional value of our food even further.

After the food is harvested, it may be stored in a warehouse for an extended period; it may even be frozen and then thawed. Fruits and vegetables lose precious vitamins and minerals when subjected to temperature changes, shipping, and storage on supermarket shelves. If you eat foods processed with lots of preservatives and synthetic additives, the nutritional value drops considerably. In our effort to make food more plentiful and cheap, we have traded good nutrition for mass-produced food with reduced nutrients and questionable quality.

Nutritional Supplementation for Health and Longevity

Given the current poor eating habits of Americans and the depletion of the nutrients in our food, nutritional supplementation is, at the very least, good "preventative health-care insurance." While nutritional supplementation provides no actual guarantees for better health, more and more scientific evidence suggests that certain nutrients may help prevent certain ailments such as diabetes, heart disease, strokes, and cancer. Even if you do put a lot of time and effort into eating nutritious meals, as I do, I still recommend taking nutritional supplements. I don't go a day without them.

Choosing Your Nutritional Supplementation

The single most important consideration when choosing a nutritional supplement is quality. The quality of the foods you eat has been severely compromised. Nutritional supplements provide you with at least one major advantage over most store-bought foods: you have the power to choose the exact level of quality you want.

I am intrigued when, as often happens, I am approached by someone who boasts about the great deal he or she got on a nutritional supplement. For heavens sake, a nutritional supplement is something that you are going to repeatedly ingest. Is this something that you want to buy based on the cheapest price? Of course you don't. Price is always a consideration, but focus on getting the best value for your dollar. While top-quality supplements may be more expensive than supplements that contain inferior and less costly ingredients and are produced by methods chosen for the sake of a cheap price, you *can* get a superior product at a reasonable price if you do your homework. While some heavily advertised name brands may have some nutritional value, be aware that much of their products' cost may be related to expensive advertising and fancy packaging rather than high-quality ingredients.

All Supplements Are Not Created Equal

When forming the foundation of your supplementation program, the best place to start is with a comprehensive multivitamin and mineral supplement. Just as if you were building a home, you want a good, solid foundation.

Modern advancements in the field of supplementation have brought some extraordinarily good products onto the market. I have taken nutritional and protein supplements for over twenty years, and I have also researched the supplement market extensively. While a wide selection is available today, it includes many more poor products. The best-quality supplements are not necessarily the ones in your local supermarket or pharmacy. Remember, many nutritional supplements are produced at the cheapest cost in order to appeal to a consumer who believes that all supplements are created equal. This is simply not the case. Why would a manufacturer spend more money producing a supplement with superior quality if these uninformed consumers are going to buy the cheapest supplement anyway? Uninformed consumers will get precisely what they ask for: lowest cost and quite possibly the lowest quality. But don't assume that the most expensive product is the best product either, because it may very well not be.

You can obtain your supplements as tablets, caplets, hard-shell or soft-shell gelatin capsules, liquids, and powdered mixes. I use comprehensive multivitamin/mineral supplements as well as protein powders with added nutrients as the foundation for my nutritional supplement program.

Quality Control Standards

Make sure your multivitamin/mineral supplement measures up to the highest standards:

- Manufactured in climate-controlled FDA-registered facilities under Federal Good Manufacturing Practices (GMPs)

- Ingredients that are tested to guarantee their identity and potency

- Manufactured to pharmaceutical standards that meet or exceed strict Federal requirements of the Dietary and Supplement Health Act (DSHEA)

- Verified for potency of ingredients and absence of pesticides, chemicals, and toxins

- Laboratory-testing of all raw materials before releasing to production

- Microbiological testing to confirm the absence of harmful bacteria, yeast, and mold

- Made to United States Pharmacopeia (USP) standards for quality, purity, and potency

- No synthetic ingredients in the coatings; preferably, made with an antioxidant coating to preserve freshness and potency

- Formulated based on valid scientific research

- Packaging that shields supplements from air and water vapor, which can degrade the active ingredients

The way supplements are manufactured can play just as important a role in the quality of the supplement as the actual ingredients. There is a tremendous difference in the manufacturing of supplements because supplement manufacturers are responsible for their own manufacturing processes; they are not required to register with the FDA or obtain FDA approval before manufacturing or selling nutritional supplements.

Ingredients to Look for in Your Multivitamin/Mineral Supplement

The quality of ingredients used in manufacturing nutritional supplements varies greatly. Because of the limited government (FDA) regulation of supplement manufacturing, it is important that you as the consumer take responsibility for knowing what's in the supplements you are buying. While supplement manufacturers are ultimately responsible for making their products safe, it is up to you to take the initiative in buying supplements that contain the highest quality of ingredients. In other words, "caveat emptor"—let the buyer beware! Remember, highest quality does not have to mean most expensive. Advertising can substantially increase production costs while adding little to the quality of the product.

Today's state-of-the-art supplements offer much more than just basic vitamin/mineral support. Here are some very important basic ingredients to look for in your search for the ideal comprehensive supplements:

- Full spectrum of water- and fat-soluble Vitamins A, C, D, E, K, and the B vitamins, including folic acid (particularly for women) and biotin

- Comprehensive minerals, including calcium, magnesium, phosphorus, iodine, potassium, selenium, molybdenum, chromium, copper, zinc, and manganese

- Trace minerals, such as silica, boron, and vanadium

- Phytonutrients (from plants), such as fruit, vegetable, and herbal extracts

- Anti-oxidant support from such substances as grape seed extract, green tea, beta-carotene, lycopene, isoflavenoids, bioflavenoids, and alpha lipoic acid

- Plant enzymes such as bromelain and papain for improved digestion

While you can get all these important nutrients and more with one nutritional supplement product, it is quite likely that full supplementation will involve more than one capsule, tablet, or serving. Also, you may choose to get your nutritional supplement foundation from more than one product.

It's important to understand that vitamins and minerals work together. You are relying on the manufacturer of the supplement to ensure that all of the nutrients are designed to work together and in the proper amounts. The dangers in attempting to combine nutritional supplements yourself are that, if you are not extremely proficient in this area, you may mix supplements that may not work well together, and you may not choose the appropriate dosages. For example, to be most beneficial to you, calcium should be taken with nutrients such as boron, phosphorus, vitamin D, and magnesium. Your supplements will be better digested and better absorbed if you take them with food. I recommend taking your supplements with both breakfast and dinner, but make sure to take them at least once daily.

A Guide to Vitamins and Minerals*

VITAMINS

A (Retinol, Carotene)

Found in liver, eggs, dark green and deep orange fruits and vegetables, dairy products
Functions: Growth and repair of body tissues, resistance to infections, bone and tooth formation, visual purple production (necessary for night vision)
Deficiency symptoms: Night blindness, drying of the eyes, dry rough skin, impaired bone growth

B-1 (Thiamin)

Found in wheat germ, liver, pork, whole grains and enriched grains, dried beans
Functions: Carbohydrate metabolism, appetite maintenance, nerve function, growth and muscle tone
Deficiency symptoms: Mental confusion, muscle weakness, edema, fatigue, loss of appetite

B-2 (Riboflavin)

Found in dairy products, leafy green vegetables, whole grains and enriched grains
Functions: Necessary for fat, carbohydrate, and protein metabolism; cell respiration, formation of antibodies
Deficiency symptoms: Sensitivity of eyes to light, cracks in corners of mouth, dermatitis around nose and lips

B-6 (Pyridoxine)

Found in fish, poultry, lean meats, whole grains
Functions: Necessary for fat, carbohydrate, and protein metabolism, and formation of antibodies
Deficiency symptoms: Dermatitis, anemia, nausea, smooth tongue

B-12 (Cyanocobalamin)

Found in organ meats, lean meat, fish, poultry, eggs, dairy products
Functions: Necessary for fat, carbohydrate, and protein metabolism; maintains healthy nervous system, aids in blood cell formation
Deficiency symptoms: Pernicious anemia, numbness and tingling in fingers and toes

Biotin

Found in egg yolks, organ meats, dark green vegetables (also made by microorganisms in the intestinal tract)
Functions: Necessary for fat, carbohydrate, and protein metabolism, formation of fatty acids; helps utilize B vitamins
Deficiency symptoms: Pale, dry scaly skin; depression; poor appetite

Folic Acid

Found in leafy green vegetables, organ meats, dried beans
Functions: Red blood cell formation, protein metabolism, growth and cell division
Deficiency symptoms: Anemia, diarrhea, smooth tongue, poor growth

* Source: www.sf.va.gov/nutrition/vitamin.htm

VITAMINS, *continued*

Niacin

Found in meat, poultry, fish, nuts, whole grains and enriched grains, dried beans
Functions: Necessary for fat, carbohydrate, and protein metabolism; health of skin, tongue, and digestive system, blood circulation
Deficiency symptoms: General fatigue, digestive disorders, irritability, loss of appetite, skin disorders

Pantothenic Acid

Found in lean meats, whole grains, legumes
Functions: Converts nutrients into energy, assists in formation of some fats, improves vitamin utilization
Deficiency symptoms: Not seen under normal circumstances (vomiting, severe abdominal cramps, fatigue, tingling hands and feet)

C (Ascorbic Acid)

Found in citrus fruits, melon, berries, vegetables
Functions: Helps heal wounds, strengthens blood vessels, maintains collagen, promotes resistance to infection
Deficiency symptoms: Bleeding gums, slow-healing wounds, easy bruising, aching joints, nosebleeds, anemia

D

Found in egg yolks, organ meats, fortified milk, also made in skin exposed to sunlight
Functions: Calcium and phosphorus metabolism (bone and teeth formation)
Deficiency symptoms: Poor bone growth, rickets, osteomalacia, muscle twitching

E (Tocopherol)

Found in vegetable oils and margarine, wheat germ, nuts, dark green vegetables, whole grains
Functions: Maintains cell membranes, protects vitamin A and essential fatty acids from oxidation, assists in red blood cell formation
Deficiency symptoms: Not seen in humans except after prolonged impairment of fat absorption (neurological abnormalities)

K

Found in leafy green vegetables, fruit, cereal, dairy products
Functions: Important in formation of blood-clotting agents
Deficiency symptoms: Tendency to hemorrhage

MINERALS

Calcium

Found in milk and milk products
Functions: Strong bones, teeth, muscle tissue; regulates heartbeat, muscle action, and nerve function, blood-clotting
Deficiency symptoms: Soft, brittle bones; back and leg pains, heart palpitations, tetany

MINERALS, *continued*

Chromium

> **Found in** brewer's yeast, cheese, whole grains, meat
> **Functions:** Glucose metabolism (energy); increases effectiveness of exercise
> **Deficiency symptoms:** Atherosclerosis, glucose intolerance in diabetics

Copper

> **Found in** oysters, nuts, organ meats, dried beans
> **Functions:** Formation of red blood cells, bone growth and health, works with vitamin C to form elastin
> **Deficiency symptoms:** Anemia, bone demineralization, nervous system disturbances

Iodine

> **Found in** seafood, iodized salt
> **Functions:** Component of the hormone thyroxine, which controls metabolism
> **Deficiency symptoms:** Goiter, obesity

Iron

> **Found in** organ meats, meat, fish, poultry, dried beans, whole grains and enriched grains, leafy green vegetables
> **Functions:** Formation of hemoglobin in blood and myoglobin in muscles that supply oxygen to cells
> **Deficiency symptoms:** Anemia (pale skin, fatigue)

Magnesium

> **Found in** nuts, green vegetables, whole grains, dried beans
> **Functions:** Enzyme activation, nerve and muscle function, calcium and potassium balance
> **Deficiency symptoms:** Nausea, muscle weakness, muscle twitching, irritability

Manganese

> **Found in** nuts, whole grains, vegetables, fruits
> **Functions:** Enzyme activation, carbohydrate and fat production, sex hormone production, skeletal development
> **Deficiency symptoms:** Abnormal bone and cartilage formation, impaired glucose tolerance

Phosphorus

> **Found in** meat, poultry, fish, eggs, dairy products, dried beans, whole grains
> **Functions:** Promotes bone development; important in protein, fat and carbohydrate utilization
> **Deficiency symptoms:** Weakness, poor appetite, bone pain

Potassium

> **Found in** vegetables, fruits, dried beans, milk, yogurt
> **Functions:** Fluid balance, controls activity of heart muscle, nervous system
> **Deficiency symptoms:** Lethargy, weakness, poor appetite, abnormal heartbeat

Protein Supplementation

My experience has been that good nutrition and a more active, fitness-oriented lifestyle go hand in hand. The more exercise you get, the more aware you are of your nutrition. As your fitness level increases, so will your need and desire for added nutritional supplementation. The more exercise you get, particularly strength training exercises, the more protein you will need. It simply takes more protein to build and repair muscles. Even if you are not yet very active (I hope you will be soon), sufficient protein intake is still important to prevent your body from cannibalizing its own muscle tissue.

Excellent sources of protein supplementation are soy, whey (derived from milk) and egg white protein. The most common form of high-quality protein supplementation is in powdered form; however, protein meal bars are also very popular. Here are some features to look for in your protein powder supplement:

- Full spectrum of amino acids, including alanine, arginine, aspartic acid, cystine, glutamine, glycine, histidine, isoleucine, leucine, lysine, methionine, ornithine, phenylalanine, proline, threonine, tryptophan, tyrosine, and valine
- Low in sugars and other carbohydrates
- No synthetic or toxic ingredients
- Good tasting

The best way to take protein in powder form is to combine various protein sources such as whey, casein (the part of milk used to make cheese), egg, and soy. Many of the protein powders on the market today already combine two or more of these different protein sources in one powder. While soy protein may not have as much protein biological value (amount of protein per serving) as some of the others, it is a super food that I strongly recommend you include in your protein supplementation. Soy protein has the highest protein value of any plant protein. Protein shakes are an excellent way to get one or more of your six meals per day.

Six Special Youth-Enhancing Supplements

Ginseng: The Longevity Herb

Ginseng as a dietary supplement is processed from the ginseng root and has become a very popular herbal remedy. Ginseng has been shown to have a number of positive health effects. There are three major forms of ginseng: American, Red Korean, and Siberian.

American Ginseng (*Panax quinquefolius*) has been found to be beneficial in a number of different ways:

- Enhances the cancer-killing power of chemotherapy drugs for breast cancer patients

- Shown to be beneficial in aiding the body's immune system's response to cancer

- Helps to moderate the effects of spikes in blood sugar levels and increased insulin as a result of eating high-glycemic index foods (such as sugar and white bread)

- Shown to be helpful for chronic fatigue and depression

- Gives women with severe menopausal symptoms improved quality of life

Red Korean Ginseng (*Panax ginseng*) has a reputation for the providing these health benefits:

- Increases energy
- Decreases sudden rise in blood pressure normally associated with an increase in stress hormones
- Relieves symptoms of asthma and other lung conditions
- Increases male and female hormone production

Siberian Ginseng, also known as *eleuthero,* is made from the dried root of *Eleuthero-coccus senticosus,* a plant native to China, Japan, Korea, and Siberia. Siberian ginseng contains compounds that favorably influence the adrenal glands, which release stress-fighting hormones. Here are some of the beneficial effects of Siberian ginseng:

- Considered a primary adaptogen, it helps in the prevention of stress-related illnesses

- Increases energy and reduces fatigue

- Helps fight fibromyalgia and chronic fatigue syndrome

- Increases nerve impulses for improved brain functioning; used to combat Alzheimer's disease

- Relieves symptoms of premenstrual syndrome (PMS)

- Increases male fertility

- Boosts the immune system; known to provide resistance for colds and flu

Studies have shown that all forms of ginseng increase strength, coordination, endurance, and muscle mass.* The quality of ginseng sold varies widely, so buy it from a reputable manufacturer. Consult your doctor before taking ginseng if you are on blood-thinning medication.

Coenzyme Q-10: Anti-aging Nutrient

A growing body of evidence from research studies (described in *Complementary Medicine,* Jan. 2002, and on the Web site ivillagehealth.com) indicates that supplementing with Coenzyme Q-10 may be beneficial in the treatment of a number of health conditions. Coenzyme Q-10 (also known as CoQ-10) is a naturally occurring nutrient found throughout your body. CoQ-10 works to produce energy in the cells of your nervous system, particularly those affecting your heart.

---

* Sources: Muscle and Fitness, September 2001; L. R. Bucci, "Selected Herbals and Human Exercise Performance," *American Journal of Clinical Nutrition,* August 2000 72 (& sup.): 6245–365.

Here are some possible health benefits of Coenzyme Q-10 supplementation:

- May retard the aging process

- Due to very powerful anti-oxidant action, may protect heart tissue from free radical damage

- May reduce the size of breast cancer tumors

- May protect against cardiomyopathy (enlarged heart), hypertension, and congestive heart failure

- Promotes healthy teeth and gums

- May improve fertility, alleviate fatigue, and improve symptoms of Alzheimer's disease

Coenzyme Q-10 supplementation certainly offers much promise in the quest for greater longevity and good health. As always, consult with your physician if you are taking pharmaceutical drugs.

Arginine: Amazing Amino Acid

Some arginine is produced by your body; however, additional supplementation can be very beneficial. Growing research on arginine is showing that this amazing amino acid has many potential benefits:

- Dilates blood vessels

- Stimulates the immune system

- Reverses affects of aging by increasing growth hormone production by the pituitary gland

- Promotes faster healing from surgery or wounds

- Increases male fertility

Arginine has another very beneficial effect: it is the substance from which creatine is made. Creatine is an amino acid that increases strength, energy, and athletic performance. I know this is true because I have used creatine myself to enhance both strength-training and aerobic workouts. Taking arginine will naturally increase the levels of creatine in your body, helping you to maximize your fitness program. I have had great personal success using a combination of 5 grams of creatine per day and 1,500 milligrams of timed-release arginine twice daily. Creatine is beneficial to both men and women.

Green Tea: Powerful Anti-oxidant

The Chinese have appreciated the powerful effects of green tea for centuries. In fact, after water, the most widely consumed beverage in the world is green tea (no, not coffee).

Green tea has one of the highest concentrations of *polyphenols* (a strong anti-oxidant) of any tea. Polyphenols have powerful cancer fighting properties. Green tea is rich in *epigallocatechin gallate* (EGCg), which has been shown to have a powerful affect on inhibiting cancer cell growth.*

Here are some of the potential benefits of green tea:

- Helps reduce incidence of heart disease and cancer

- Has youth-enhancing characteristics; good for protection of skin and organs

- Helps with digestion and may protect against ulcers

- May be beneficial for the immune system

- Inhibits formation of bacteria and viruses

---

* See Z. P. Chen et al., "Green Tea epigallocatechin gallate shows a pronounced growth inhibitory effect on cancerous cells but not on their normal counterparts," *Cancer Letters* 1998, 173–79, and Marissa Melton, "The Power of Tea: Component Identified That Inhibits Cancer," *U.S. News and World Report,* Dec. 1998, p. 58.

Green tea is not "the only game in town." A tea called *rooibos* (pronounced roy-boss), made from the South African shrub *aspalathus linearis,* shows great promise. Rooibus tea offers 50% more anti-oxidant protection than green tea and, unlike green tea, is naturally caffeine-free.

While some of the effects claimed by green tea and rooibos tea have yet to be proven, growing evidence points to great health benefits. In addition, these teas can offer you a very relaxing and good tasting beverage to help you unwind after a productive and positive day.

Calcium and Magnesium: Dynamic Duo of Supplements

Calcium is the most abundant mineral in your body. It is vital that you have enough calcium to ensure strong bones and teeth. Magnesium, a mineral that many are deficient in, is a close partner to calcium, and together they work in synergy to create the following health benefits:

- Support bone health, especially for menopausal women, and help prevent osteoporosis

- Promote sound sleep

- Reduce muscle cramps and menstrual cramps

Magnesium has been shown to relax blood vessels; this effect could be beneficial in preventing heart disease. In addition, magnesium works with the body's enzymes to digest food.

Calcium and magnesium are important nutrients for everyone. However, if you are pregnant, lactating, or postmenopausal, your calcium/magnesium needs are greater. A word of caution however about calcium supplements. A University of Florida (Gainesville) study (*Journal of the American Medical Association,* Sept. 2000) found that eight of 22 calcium supplements tested contained lead. Choose your supplements wisely; *never* accept calcium supplements containing lead.

Glucosamine for Healthy Joints

There are 76,000,000 "baby boomers" in the United States, and one-third of the baby-boomer population is over 50 years of age. As the baby boomers (and their parents) get older, a major health concern faces them all—joint problems. As we age, the amount of cushioning cartilage in our joints declines. This results in a progressive narrowing of the joint space, which can result in pain, stiffness, and a decline in joint function and mobility. Arthritis can develop if joint integrity continues to decline.

Fortunately there is help. Glucosamine is the building block for ligaments, tendons, and fluid in the joints. It also gives cartilage strength, structure, and resiliency. Glucosamine is now commonly used as a nutritional supplement to promote healthy joint functioning throughout life and is often combined with other nutrients to further increase its efficiency. These are some of the beneficial ingredients used in conjunction with glucosamine:

- Chondroitin, prevalent in connective tissues

- Methosulfonylmethane (MSM), the best source of bio-available, organic sulfur, to offer nutritional support for joint functioning

- Ginger extract and alpinia galanga to help promote mobility of the joints

Herbal Adaptogens: Turbo-Charge Your Health

In today's technologically advanced society we are constantly bombarded by many different forms of stress that can harm our health and well-being. The three major sources of stress are environmental, physiological (body), and psychological (mind).

Environmental stress. The environment bombards us with a variety of stressors: pollutants from automobiles, boats, and airplanes; industrial waste; tobacco smoke (including second hand smoke); pesticides and synthetic chemicals in the water, air, and food. In addition, increased solar radiation from the depleted ozone layer, as well as nuclear catastrophes like Three Mile Island and Chernobyl and petrochemical disasters like the Exxon *Valdez* accident, place enormous stress on us.

Physiological stress. This includes stresses placed on our bodies. Examples include poor diet, lack of adequate nutritional supplementation, aging, lack of sleep, poor physical fitness, PMS and menopause in women, and illness.

Psychological stress emanates from our thoughts. Examples of situations that cause psychological stress include commuting to and from your job in rush hour traffic, going through marital problems and divorce, the illness or death of a loved one, studying for an exam, anxiety, and depression.

Regardless of which form or forms of stress you are enduring, your mind and body are integrated as one, and what effects one part of you ultimately effects your entire being. All of the stresses we face are compounded by the lightning speed with which the world changes today due to technological, business, personal and societal factors. These rapid and constant changes force us to *adapt* very quickly to the changes confronting us.

A variety of health problems are associated with our inability to adapt to the stresses placed upon us by the environment, our bodies, and our minds:

- PMS in women

- Decreased sexual functioning in both men and women

- Acceleration of the aging process and the higher incidence of disease that this brings

- Decrease in human growth hormone excreted by the pituitary gland

- Diseases of the digestive tract including ulcers, nausea and gastric cancer

- Overeating and resulting obesity as a response to stress

- Chronic fatigue syndrome

- Suppressed immune functioning leading to serious illness

- Various forms of cancer which tend to develop at the site of the stressed area (e.g. smokers developing lung cancer)

In fact, stress has been linked to most diseases and ailments in one way or another. In addition to the health problems caused by stress, another extremely important factor to consider about stress is the potential it has to negatively impact your entire lifestyle. For the many people who are unable to cope with stress, life can be a struggle filled with little happiness, joy, or achievement. Don't let it happen to you!

There is a great deal you can do about the negative stress that bombards you every day. One of the most important discoveries ever made concerning our ability to adapt to the stresses and changes in our lives occurred in Russia beginning in 1951. At that time numerous research studies (many of which have not been translated into English) begun by the U.S.S.R. Academy of Science uncovered the secret to adaptation to stress—*adaptogens.*

Adaptogens are natural herbs (preferably synergistically formulated) that help the body cope with internal and external stressors. Adaptogens are unique in their ability to maintain homeostasis within your body, creating a state of *internal balance.* If you are tired, adaptogens work to improve your mental functioning and physical endurance. If you are exercising or physically active, adaptogens help to improve stamina and assist your body in building muscle tissue.

Herbal adaptogens can help you in many ways. Here are some of the many health benefits associated with herbal adaptogens:

- Increases metabolism to burn fat

- Builds bone marrow and muscle tissue

- Maintains normal blood pressure and cholesterol levels

- Contains anti-aging properties to help you look and feel younger

- Helps body to utilize oxygen most efficiently

- Supports healthy heart and circulatory system

- Improves mental functioning and athletic performance

- Inhibits free-radical (cancer-causing) damage

- Improves sleep

- Supports major organs, including liver, kidneys, and heart

- Promotes a healthy immune system by supporting infection resistance and recovery

As with nutritional supplements, all types of herbal adaptogen formulas are available. The formulas of some herbal adaptogens include only one or two essential herbs. Newer, more comprehensive adaptogen formulas contain a variety of synergistically blended herbs plus additional natural plant products for maximum adaptogen benefits.

I suggest that you look for the following ingredients when selecting an herbal adaptogen:

- *Schizandra,* a seed extract, supports central nervous system and liver functioning plus improves night vision.

- *Rhodiola* helps to eliminate toxic chemicals, increase oxygen utilization, reduce stress, and activate DNA repair.

- *Licorice, cordyceps mushroom,* and *elderberry* help protect you from free-radical damage by stimulating natural killer cells.

- *American ginseng* maintains blood sugar levels, fights chronic fatigue, and reduces PMS symptoms.

- *Reishi mushrooms,* used in Chinese medicine, restore internal balance and support immune system functioning as well as resistance to stress.

- *Siberian ginseng* maintains normal blood pressure and cholesterol levels for those in the normal range. In addition, it increases energy, helps relieve PMS, and improves sexual functioning.

- *Korean ginseng* decreases stress-hormone production and improves respiratory function.

Additional beneficial ingredients to look for in your herbal adaptogen include fresh ashwagandha root, pantocrene, fresh milky oats seed, green tea, grape seed and skin, hawthorn, and ginger root.

As with any of your nutritional supplements, look for exceptional quality of ingredients and manufacturing processes. Seek out a company whose primary concern is providing exceptional products and helping people live healthier lives, rather than a company that uses nutritional supplements primarily to maximize its corporate profits. While extremely rare, such companies and people do exist today.

Human Growth Hormones: War on Aging

With the 85+ age group becoming the fastest growing segment of the population, and with one baby boomer turning 50 about every eight seconds, there is growing interest in human growth hormones as a way to literally turn back the hands of time.

Dr. Ronald Klatz is one of the world's leading growth hormone experts and President of the American Academy of Anti-aging Medicine. According to Dr. Klatz, "By replenishing your supply of growth hormone, you can recover your vigor, health, looks, and sexuality. For the first time in human history, we can intervene in the aging process, restore many aspects of youth, resist disease, substantially improve the quality of life, and perhaps extend the life span itself. The 'fountain of youth' lies within the cells of each of us. All you need to do is release it."

Human growth hormone is the most abundant hormone made by the pituitary gland. As we age, human growth hormone levels naturally decline, and many in the scientific community believe that this decline in growth hormone production is one of the primary reasons we age. According to recent growth-hormone research, low levels of growth hormone are now associated with a higher incidence of disease and shorter life spans. Of great importance, however, is the growing body of research showing that human growth hormones may prevent or possibly even reverse many diseases of our time and the degenerative effects of aging.

Here are some beneficial health effects that increased growth hormone levels offer:

- Strengthened immune system and possible assistance in the fight against some cancers

- Improved and restored lung capacity

- Reversal of heart disease

- Increased bone mass

- Increased energy, faster metabolism, and greater weight loss

- Improved sexual function

- More youthful appearance; particularly helpful to the skin and hair

Increasing our levels of growth hormone may retard and possibly even reverse the aging process. The big problem with traditional growth hormone replacement therapy injections are that they are extremely expensive and can have potentially dangerous side effects, as have some prescription drugs that are used to increase growth hormone levels.

There is another solution, a "natural" way to raise growth hormone levels: you can follow an all-natural program designed to help your pituitary gland release growth hormones into your bloodstream. Here are some important steps you can take to raise your growth hormones naturally, inexpensively, and without harmful side effects.

—*Eight Steps to Increased Longevity*—

Step 1: Drink more water.

Drink at least 8 ounces (1 cup) of water for every 20 pounds of body weight. I weigh 204 pounds, so I drink at least ten 8-ounce glasses a day. (Soda, coffee, alcohol, and tea do not count as water intake.)

Step 2: Eat a balanced diet.

Eat a whole food diet with plenty of low-glycemic fruits and vegetables (see my recommended list on page 168). Eat six smaller meals per day instead of a few big ones.

Step 3: Eat more lean protein.

Eat lean protein foods and supplement your diet with nutritious protein shakes and protein food bars. The amino acids arginine, glutamine, and lysine are particularly important, so be sure your protein supplement contains generous amounts of them.

Step 4: Supplement your vitamin and mineral intake.

Take top-quality vitamin/mineral supplements that include:

- A full spectrum vitamin/mineral profile
- Phytonutrients such as plant enzymes, fruit and vegetable extracts, herbal and green food extracts
- Complete anti-oxidant support
- Trace minerals
- Coenzyme Q-10

Step 5: Exercise.

Do some form of aerobic exercise and/or strength training at least five days a week. Studies have shown that strength training is far superior to aerobic exercise in releasing growth hormones. In addition, you will get a certain feeling and a more sculpted look from strength training that you cannot get from aerobic exercises. Strength training increases muscle size as well as bone mass. It helps protect your joints, especially if you prefer aerobic exercises, which are tough on the joints. In addition to releasing growth hormones, exercising will help you look and feel better and give you added confidence as well as a more positive outlook on life.

Step 6: Make positive connections.

There are tremendous benefits to having fulfilling relationships with loved ones and friends. Laughing together is very beneficial to mind, body, and soul alike. Consider watching a comedy such as *Captain Ron* (with Martin Short), *Overboard* (Goldie Hawn and Kurt Russell), or *What About Bob?* (Bill Murray and Richard Dreyfus) with someone special. Just experience the moment and observe how good it feels. Laughter is both exhilarating and relaxing at the same time. It's wonderful anti-aging medicine. Cultivate positive relationships to help each other live longer, healthier lives.

Step 7: Indulge in nature and sunshine.

Emory University's Rollins School of Public health researcher's suggest that being out in nature can be uplifting and healthy. I'm certain of it. Going for a hike in the woods or strolling along the seashore is inherently beneficial. Breathing fresh air is rejuvenating. Get outside for at least a half an hour a day, and strive to spend at least fifteen minutes of it in the sun, even if it means just taking a stroll around the block at lunchtime or after work. It's also fulfilling to go outside at night and just gaze up at the moon and stars. Being out in nature gives us a certain spiritual connection, a feeling of being in tune with the vast universe. The positive feelings we gain from this experience will contribute in a big way towards greater longevity. Take the necessary steps to increase your potential for greater longevity and happiness. It's all within your control!

Step 8: Get plenty of sleep.

Get eight hours of sleep per night. Sleep is crucial to increasing your growth hormone levels. Many Americans are sleep-deprived, and this contributes greatly to their premature aging. If you have trouble sleeping, try the natural hormone *melatonin.*

—*The Road Back to a Good Night's Sleep*—

"It is better to sleep on things beforehand than lie awake
thinking about them afterwards."
Baltasar Gracian

It is estimated that 100 million Americans have problems sleeping. In 2001 the National Sleep Foundation, a nonprofit organization studying sleep and sleep disorders, reported that:

- One-third of Americans are working more and getting less sleep now than five years ago.

- Two thirds of Americans get less than eight hours of sleep a night.

- One half of all American adults drive while drowsy.

The National Highway Traffic Safety Administration says that at least 100,000 traffic accidents per year occur due to sleepy drivers and 40,000 people are injured, 1,550 fatally. A lack of sleep can also cause serious health problems, such as high blood pressure, heart disease, and strokes. Sleeplessness also weakens the immune system, leaving you more vulnerable to viruses and bacteria.

If that weren't enough, a 2001 Sleep in America Poll surveying 1,004 adults reported the following:

- 43% of Americans use caffeine to stay awake, and 5% use stronger stimulants to avoid falling asleep.

- 52% of Americans spent less time having sex than five years ago, and 38% have sex less than once a week.

- Among married adults having trouble sleeping, a whopping 77% reported less marital satisfaction.

Sleep disorders reported in the study were disturbingly common: 9% reported sleep apnea, a serious breathing disorder in which a sleeper can stop breathing for as long as two minutes; 13% had restless legs syndrome; and 38% snored.

It's pretty clear that we Americans as a group get very low grades for sleep. It's also very clear that sleep is absolutely essential. Sleep deprivation is known to reduce the release of human growth hormones, which may partly explain the terrible feeling we get after not getting a good night's sleep.

Because a good night's sleep is so vitally important to achieving your desired lifestyle, fitness level, and goals, it's important that you use all the sleep-enhancing tools at your disposal. Here are the six steps to a good night's sleep:

Six Steps to a Good Night's Sleep

Step 1: Lose weight.

Researchers at Monash University in Melbourne, Australia, report that weight reduction cuts snoring by as much as 68% (your sleep partner will appreciate that) and improves overall sleep quality by 37% . Maintaining your proper weight will of course improve many other areas of your life as well.

Step 2: Develop a regular sleep pattern.

Establish regular times for going to sleep and waking up. The idea that it's good to "sleep in" on weekends is faulty for several reasons. If you are getting enough sleep, you shouldn't need to alter your sleep pattern even on the weekends. When you adopt the habit of a regular sleep pattern, you will also notice a reduced reliance on your alarm clock. If commuting to and from work is costing you valuable sleep (and good health) seriously consider working from a home office. (Refer to Chapter 3, "The Home-Based Business Revolution.")

Step 3: Develop an ideal sleep environment.

In order to have a good sleeping environment you don't have to be like the Conehead family in the old Saturday Night Live skits and create a "sleep chamber." Instead, make sure the room is cool; this will simulate your body's reduced internal temperature. Also, make sure the room is as dark and quiet as possible. If you live in the city, you may find wearing an eye mask or earplugs beneficial. Sleeping out in the country with the sound of crickets always helps me get a good night's sleep. Finally, make sure you have a good, comfortable bed.

Step 4: Avoid stimulants and alcohol.

Caffeine—found in coffee, tea, and soda—is a stimulant that has a cumulative effect on your body over the course of a day. Caffeine can actually stay in your system for as long as twelve hours. Try to limit your caffeine intake, and don't take any after noon.

Nicotine found in cigarettes is also a stimulant. Smokers find it more difficult to fall asleep and wake up, and they experience withdrawal symptoms during the night. Hopefully, if you are still smoking, the health habits you will adopt by reading this book will help you give it up for good. The better you feel about your body and yourself, the less you will want to smoke.

Even though alcohol is a depressant and may cause you to fall asleep initially, it will cause you to wake up repeatedly during the night. Alcohol can also cause nightmares and snoring, and may lead to sleep apnea. Depressants such as alcohol interfere with REM (rapid eye movement) sleep, the period of deep sleep when dreaming occurs. Less REM sleep typically results in more restless sleep with more frequent awakenings. A glass of "heart healthy" red wine at dinner is fine, but don't overdo it if you want a good night's sleep. Never take sleeping pills and alcohol together.

Step 5: Have a light bedtime snack.

Heavy meals close to bedtime will interfere with sleep (heavy meals are a bad idea in general). A light bedtime snack of carbohydrates such as whole-grain breads or cereal will trigger the release of seratonin, a natural sleep inducer. Also, foods containing L-Tryptophan, such as milk or turkey, will also facilitate sleep. If you stick to a healthy balanced diet of six smaller meals per day, you will not feel the need to overeat at bedtime.

Step 6: Exercise and relieve stress.

In a Stanford University study, healthy adults with minor sleep problems who exercised just forty minutes twice a week fell asleep more quickly and slept an additional forty-five minutes than those with no exercise. Exercise is a natural stress reliever, but any exercise should be completed at least four hours before bedtime. I suggest exercising a minimum of five days per week.

It's a good idea to engage in some "winding down" activity to relax before bedtime. A hot bath or twenty minutes in a jacuzzi does wonders to relax tense muscles. Relaxing your mind is equally important. I find that writing down all the things that need to be accomplished the next day helps relieve my mind before sleep. Also, avoid reading anything "work-related" before bedtime. Instead use mental imagery to think of something both pleasurable and relaxing at the same time.

As your lifestyle becomes increasingly fitness and nutritionally oriented, the quality and quantity of your sleep will dramatically improve. You will look and feel better, as well as think more clearly.

A Guide to Body Mass Index (BMI)

What is the Body Mass Index?

- BMI is a measure of weight in relation to height.

How can you figure out your BMI?

- Go to Web site www.nhlbi.nih.gov/guidelines/obesity/bmi_tbl.htm, where you can locate your height and weight, or
- Calculate it yourself, using this formula:

$$BMI = \left\{ \frac{\text{weight in pounds}}{\text{height in inches}^2} \right\} \times 703$$

1. Multiply your height (in inches) times itself.
2. Divide your weight in pounds by the result from step one.
3. Multiply your answer in step two by 703.

For example, here are the calculations for a woman who is five feet five inches tall and weighs 140 pounds:

1. *Five feet five inches is 65 inches. 65 x 65 = 4225*
2. *140 divided by 4225 = 0.0331*
3. *0.0331 x 703 = 23.27*

What is the significance of BMI?

The NIH (National Institutes of Health) has determined that, *in adults* (20 and older), a healthy weight is 18.5–24.9 on the BMI. People with a BMI of 25.0–29.9 may be classified as overweight. A BMI of 30 and above could indicate obesity.

BMI correlates well with total body fat for most people. However, keep in mind that BMI has some limitations. For instance, it can overestimate body fat in persons who are very muscular, and it can underestimate body fat in persons who have lost muscle mass, such as many elderly people. *An actual diagnosis of overweight or obesity should be made by a health professional.*

The NIH recommends the following:

- If you are overweight or obese, losing just 10% of your body weight can improve your health.
- If you need to lose weight, do so gradually—one half to two pounds per week.
- Stay physically active to balance the calories you consume.

For more information on this topic, visit the Web site:

surgeongeneral.gov/topics/obesity/calltoaction/fact_advice.htm

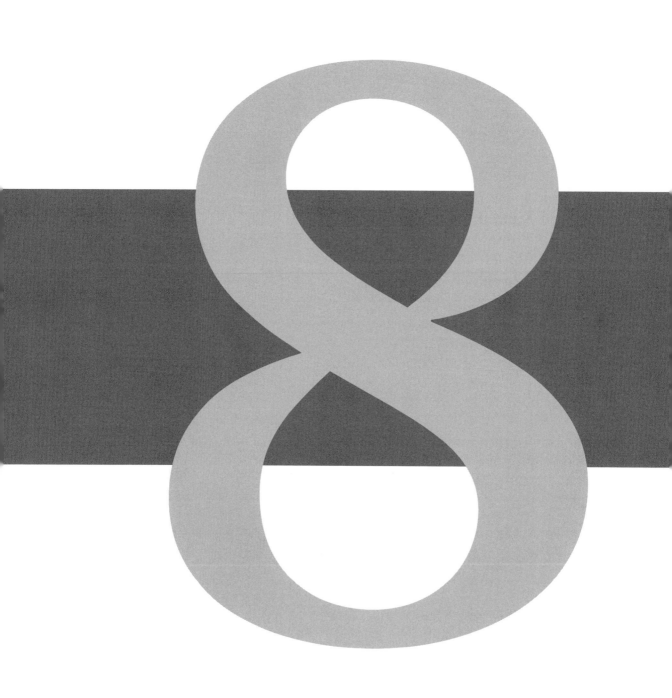

CHAPTER EIGHT

Building a Better Body

Building a Better Body

Open your mind completely to a new you!
Your body will take on the look you've imagined.

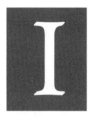

've got an interesting proposition for you. Before I make this proposition, however, I will ask only one thing of you: to consider my plan with a *completely* open mind, placing no limitations whatsoever upon yourself. My proposal is that from this day forward you will begin to see yourself as having the type of body you've always wanted. That's right, think of what you would like to look like at this very moment.

Hold that picture in your imagination. How would it make you feel to look your best? How would it make you feel to look fabulous in the types of clothes you like to wear, like that bathing suit you've always wanted? The answer is that it would make you feel great! It's time you took me up on my proposition. It's never too late to look and feel your best.

So tell me, how does the thought of having the body you've always wanted *really* make you feel right now? Before you jump to any conclusions (remember you're approaching this with an open mind), I am not necessarily suggesting that you should strive to look like the Incredible Hulk or Arnold Schwarzenegger. What I *am* suggesting is that you start thinking about how a more sculpted and fit body would make you think and feel. Strength training is something that you can start doing immediately to begin improving your fitness level and body shape.

You should always consult with a physician
before beginning an exercise or fitness program.

—Believe It and Achieve It—

Anything you want or aspire to in life begins as a single thought regardless of whether or not you actually believe that thought. As your subconscious mind begins to recognize this thought as being attainable, it will then become reality. Get rid of any limiting thoughts you have about your ability to sculpt your body. No matter what your body shape and fitness levels are today, you can improve them, and I'll show you how.

Some of the most inspiring acts of bravery and athleticism I have ever seen are performed by the physically and mentally challenged kids who compete in the Special Olympics. The example of the Special Olympics, one we can all use in our daily lives, is to start from where we are today, believe we can accomplish our goal, and move towards that goal in some way every day. The goal of looking your best and becoming more fit and healthy is one of the best things you can do for yourself. Set your "better body goal" right now. Review the Five Steps to Success in Chapter 1, "A Fantastic Voyage," and apply these principles to building the body you really want!

—Benefits of Strength Training—

During the 1970s, 1980s, and much of the 1990s, aerobic exercise was the rage. Aerobics and jazzercise classes in health clubs became a fad. High impact progressed to low impact, and the beat went on. I have been involved in some form of strength training for as long as I can remember; as a very young child, I worked out with Mom in front of the TV watching Jack LaLanne, the fabulous fitness trainer.

Certainly, some form of aerobic exercise such as walking, cycling, swimming, or jogging should be a part of every fitness program. However, since the mid 1990s, the many benefits of strength training and bodybuilding are becoming more apparent to more people every day. Many of the fitness classes in today's health clubs incorporate weight training in their routines. In addition, myths regarding bodybuilding are being dispelled. When I first began strength training as an athlete more than 20 years ago, bodybuilding was very much misunderstood. Bodybuilders were thought of as being somewhat unusual, and female bodybuilders were virtually nonexistent. Today women no longer fear becoming muscle-bound; they understand that most women would have difficulty achieving that muscle-bound look even if they *wanted* to look that way. It would be extremely difficult for most women to acquire the large muscles you see on women in the bodybuilding magazines—to do so would require many, many hours a day in the gym (besides having the right genes).

Bodybuilding is something you do to enhance the way you look, the way you feel about yourself, and even the way you think. Whether you want to develop large muscles or just get your body better toned and sculpted, the choice is yours. You get to create the look you want, like an artist painting a picture. That's part of the beauty of it: with bodybuilding you get to carry around your work of art everywhere you go, feeling great about your accomplishment. In addition to making you look and feel better, strength training can give you many other health benefits.

According to a landmark study by the American Heart Association ("Circulation," *Journal of the American Heart Association,* 2/2000), "Weight training can lower the risk of having a heart attack or stroke by lowering the LDL 'bad' cholesterol and raising the HDL 'good' cholesterol. Weight training also helps to reduce blood pressure." Weight training can also reduce the possibility of your developing diabetes by improving your body's metabolism of sugar.

Weight training increases metabolism by adding muscle. One advantage of weight lifting over aerobics is that you are building bigger muscles, which will provide a more prolonged increase in metabolism for longer periods of time. This will not only help you lose weight but also will help you develop a better shape.

Research concerning the beneficial effects of strength training have been going on for quite some time. One of the most significant studies was conducted in 1994: Tufts University's Human Nutrition Research Center on Aging conducted a 10-week strength-training exercise study on a group of men and women aged 63 to 98, in which 83% of the group required a cane, wheelchair, or walker and 66% of the group had fallen within the past year. Each participant in the study took part in an intensive strength-training program that included strenuous leg-press strength-training exercises three times per week. During the 10-week study, incredible results were reported, including significant gains in muscle size as well as improvements in strength, stability, and stamina. Many people in the study group discarded their walkers and, in some cases, improved enough to require only a cane.

Here are some additional health benefits associated with exercise and strength training:

- Improved posture
- Relief from or elimination of back pain
- Reduced incidence of depression
- Enhanced sexual pleasure
- Increased bone mass
- Decreased likelihood of injury
- Reduced risk of osteoporosis
- Stronger muscles, tendons, and ligaments
- Stronger immune system
- Deeper and longer sleep
- Reduced risk of glaucoma
- Improved short-term memory
- Reduced risk of some cancers
- Improved digestion
- Increased growth-hormone levels
- Improved self-esteem and self-image

In addition, strength training is an excellent way to lift your spirits and attain a more positive and youthful outlook on life—to simply feel better about yourself.

Strength Training as Your Foundation

One indisputable fact about fitness is that, without sufficient strength in your muscles, tendons, and ligaments, you literally could not stand up or function in any way. There-fore, ensuring that your body is strong will allow you to be healthier longer than you might have previously thought possible. Strong muscles are also good for your joints; and strong joints, in turn, can help you play your favorite sports such as tennis or golf at a higher performance level for more years.

—*Total Fitness*—

As marvelous as strength training is, it is only one component of a complete fitness regimen, as represented by the Fitness Triangle on page 234. In order to have "total" fitness you should also incorporate some form of aerobic exercise into your fitness program. Aerobic literally means "with oxygen" referring to exercise that improves cardiovascular and respiratory health. Walking, jogging, swimming, snow skiing and cycling are common aerobic exercises.

Fat-Burning Exercises

According to the American Council on Exercise, the following recommended activities burn the greatest number of calories per minute (listed in order from most calories burned to the least):

- Running at an 8 minutes per mile (mpm) pace
- Jogging at a 10 mpm pace
- Swimming at a moderate pace
- Basketball
- Weight training
- Golf (without cart)
- Walking
- Tennis
- Cycling at 10 miles per hour (mph)
- Hiking

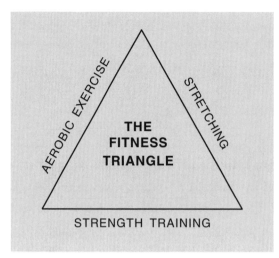

While strength training does provide some degree of cardiovascular benefit, aerobic exercise provides additional benefits and should be used as an important part of your fitness program.

Here are some tips regarding your aerobic conditioning:

• Make sure you enjoy your aerobic workout. If it's drudgery, you won't do it well nor do it for long.

• Try getting in your aerobic workout outdoors in a natural setting. If you enjoy the beach, walk or run along the water. If you prefer the mountains or woods, go hiking in the fresh air.

• If you have a slower metabolism, aerobic exercise should be a bigger part of your fitness program than the program of someone with a faster metabolism.

• You don't need to run a marathon to get a good aerobic workout: 30 minutes three times a week is sufficient, provided you are actually exercising for the entire 30 minutes.

Studies have shown that exercising on an empty stomach will help you lose weight faster, if losing weight is your goal. In addition, there is strong evidence that exercising in the morning is more efficient for burning fat. However, the main point is that you get your aerobic exercise. For me, the morning, especially when I just wake up is not a time when I want to go running on the beach (my favorite). However, I do like doing my sit-ups shortly after I awake. Exercise at a time you like, and make it work to suit your lifestyle. Again, if you force yourself to exercise at a specific time that doesn't feel right for you, eventually you will give it up. Your goal should be to find a reason to fit in your workout, not find reasons to skip your workout. It's all about establishing a habit of working out. When you do that, you are well on your way to being fit for life.

Strive to make your aerobic workouts fun as well as challenging. Change your aerobic workout occasionally to avoid stagnating. If you like to walk, consider taking a different route, or go with a friend or your dog. Keep what you do fresh and new. Be creative with your aerobic exercising so that you stay mentally and physically fit and refreshed. Listening to your favorite music can also be both motivating and inspiring.

Six Steps to Effective Aerobic Training

As with any form of exercise, your first priority is injury prevention. Therefore, always take the following steps when getting your aerobic exercise:

Step 1: Warm-up

Warm up slowly by performing at low intensity for several minutes. Your warm-up exercise does not have to be the same as your aerobic activity.

Step 2: Light Stretching

After a short warm-up, do a light stretch of the muscles involved.

Step 3: Progressively Increase Intensity

After stretching, gradually build up to a more strenuous level of exercise.

Step 4: Challenge Yourself

Move into the challenging part of your aerobic exercise where you push yourself a bit more than you did during your previous workout. Do not be concerned about what others are doing—this is *your* workout, and what is currently a challenge to you has absolutely nothing to do with what is challenging to someone else. Your challenge is simply doing a little more than your previous workout, even if that only means taking one more step than you did last time.

Step 5: Downshift

Begin to gradually reduce your level of intensity and shift into the "cool down" phase of your workout. Never stop your exercising "cold," but instead "downshift"— much as the transmission of a car goes from fourth gear to third, down to second, and then eventually to first. Downshifting should also take several minutes.

Step 6: Cool Down

Begin the cool-down phase of your routine. Lightly stretch the muscles you have used during your workout to maintain flexibility and increase blood flow to the muscles involved.

Always drink water before, during, and after your aerobic workout. Most importantly, have fun!

—Stretching—

I am amazed at how little attention and respect is paid to one of the three primary components of the Fitness Triangle. Just like Rodney Dangerfield, the guy who gets no respect, stretching is the "get no respect" part of fitness. However, stretching is a crucial part of your fitness program for several important reasons. Here are some of them:

Four Good Reasons for Stretching

1. Stretching prevents injury.

When you suddenly move parts of your body past their normal range of motion or lift an object heavier than you normally would, particularly in an awkward manner, you are increasing the possibility of trauma to muscles, ligaments, and tendons. Stretching can develop the additional flexibility to reduce or prevent injury.

2. Stretching helps you achieve your full range of motion.

Any exercises, particularly strength training exercises, are more effective and beneficial when performed through a full range of motion. Without including stretching in your fitness routine, you will probably never achieve the complete range of motion you are capable of. As an example, when performing the bench presses for the chest, many bodybuilders never achieve the full range of motion they could have. Simple chest-stretching exercises during your chest routine can help increase your range of motion, which ultimately results in stronger and larger muscles. In addition, exercising using a full range of motion reduces your chance of injury.

3. Stretching makes you stronger.

Yes, it's true: stretching between strength training "sets" (groups of exercises) can make you stronger. In a study monitored by Wayne Westcott, Ph.D., of the South Shore YMCA in Quincy, Massachusetts (described in *Men's Fitness,* 7/2001) subjects who followed a 10-week program of 20-second stretches following completion of weight-lifting sets gained 10% more strength on average than those who did not stretch. While results like these can vary dramatically from person to person, I can personally attest to the strength gains I have experienced as a result of stretching between weight training sets.

4. Stretching assists with fascia breakout.

Fascia is the ultra-strong tissue encasing your muscles. The fascia can bind muscles so strongly that muscle growth is inhibited. The fascia works somewhat like steel belts on radial tires, encasing the muscles and holding them tightly in place. Stretching after exercising or after a strength-training movement helps the muscle slowly break free of the rigid fascia casing and allows it to grow to its full potential. There is ample evidence to support the notion that a warmed-up muscle has greater potential for expansion than a cold muscle. Therefore, it is natural to conclude that the best time to stretch for maximum growth is when the muscle has been engaged in strength training or some other form of exercise.

Stretching Tips

- Always perform a warm-up exercise—such as walking, light weight-lifting, cycling, or rowing—*before* stretching.

- Many of us were taught to do stretches that we now know can cause damage to the joints, ligaments, and nerves. Similar damage can result when stretches are performed incorrectly. Perform *only* those stretches that won't cause harm, and always perform them using proper form.

- It is important to remember that stretching should not be a timed event. The idea that you must hold your stretch for 20 seconds is a faulty notion. Stretch until a mild tension in the muscle is gone. Do not force the stretch—and no pain should be present.

Stretching Exercises

The following stretching exercises will help you increase your flexibility, range of motion, strength, and muscle size while reducing your chance for injury. These stretches were selected specifically because they put minimal pressure on the ligaments, joints, and connective tissue. The exercises are grouped by individual body parts.

LOWER
BACK

Knee to Chest

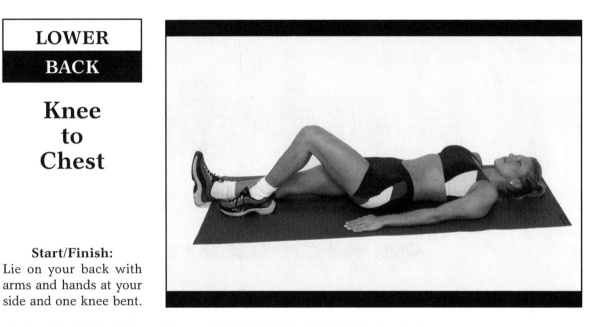

Start/Finish:
Lie on your back with arms and hands at your side and one knee bent.

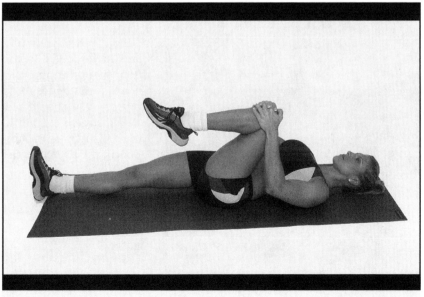

The Stretch:
Grab and hold the bent knee with both hands clasped. Pull knee toward your chest and feel the stretch. Repeat with your other leg.

LOWER

BACK

Spinal "T" Stretch

Start/Finish:
Lie on your back with your arms out, forming a "T," with palms facing up, feet flat on the floor, and knees bent.

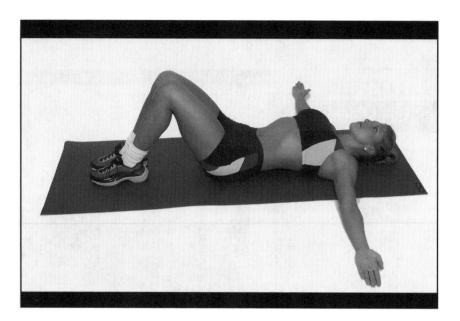

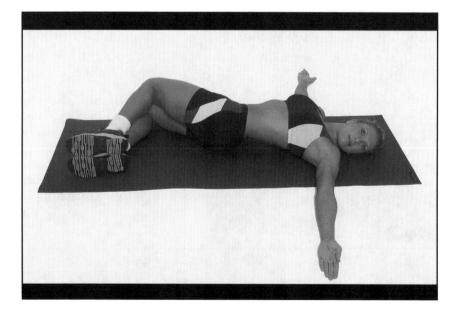

The Stretch:
Slowly lower your legs and lower body to the floor while turning your head in the opposite direction. You should feel a mild stretch but not to the point of any pain. Repeat the stretch to the other side.

Gluteus Maximus Stretch

The gluteus maximus is also known as the "glutes" or buttocks.

GLUTEUS
MAXIMUS

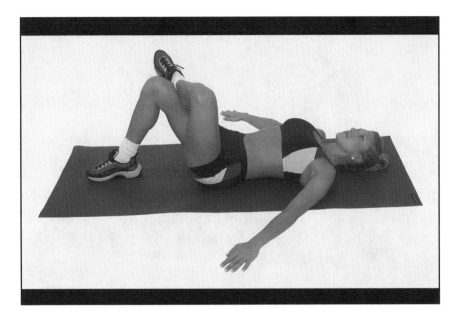

Start/Finish:
Lie on your back with arms outstretched and palms down. Put one foot flat on the floor with knee bent and cross the other leg over the knee of your bent leg.

The Stretch:
Use your hands to lift leg by grasping leg beneath the knee. Lift your leg and feel the stretch in the gluteus maximus and hip. Do not pull too hard. Repeat to the other side. (You may use a towel to assist if this makes it easier.)

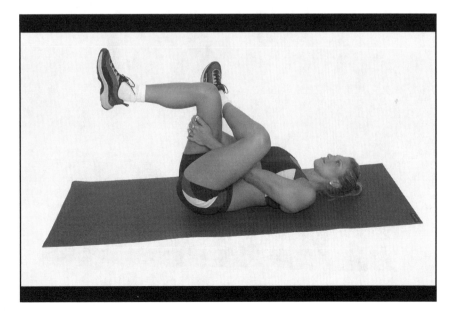

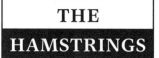

The hamstring muscles are located behind your thighs. Stretching the hamstrings is extremely important, not only to protect the hamstrings themselves, but also to reduce the risk of lower back injury.

Hamstring Isolation Stretch

Start/Finish:
This is my favorite hamstring stretch. Lying on your back, extend one leg straight out. Lift your other leg about three-fourths of the way up and place an elastic band or towel in the arch of that foot.

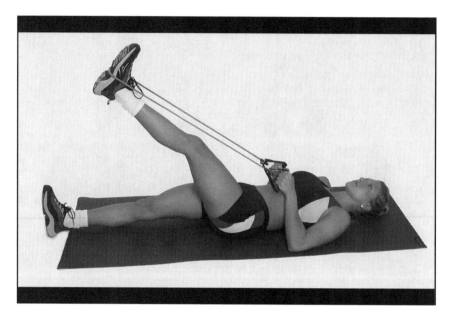

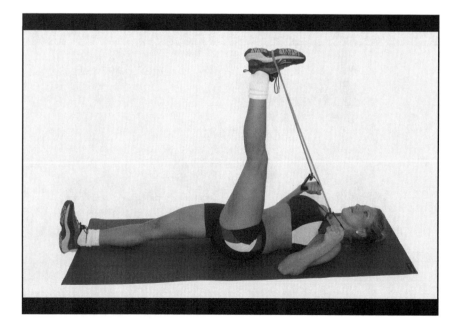

The Stretch:
Pull your raised leg towards you while keeping the leg as straight as possible. (It is perfectly acceptable to bend your knee slightly, and you should not experience any pain.) This stretch isolates the hamstrings better than any other hamstring stretch I have tried. In addition, it reduces weight-bearing stress on tendons and ligaments of the spine, hips, and pelvis.

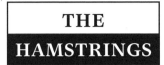

THE HAMSTRINGS

Seated Hamstring Stretch

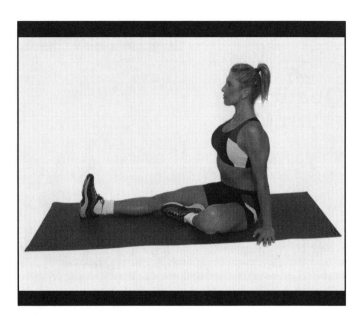

Start/Finish:
Sit on the floor in an upright position, back straight with arms supporting your upper body. Extend one leg out straight with your opposing leg bent and the bottom of your foot resting against the thigh of your extended leg.

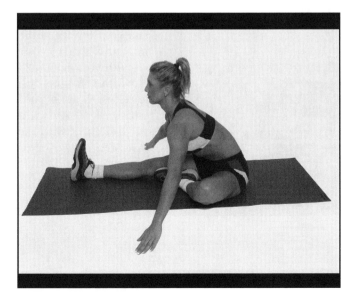

The Stretch:
Lean forward until you experience a mild stretch in your hamstring. Repeat with the other leg.

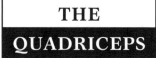

The quadriceps (also known as "quads")
are your thigh muscles.

Lying Quadriceps Stretch

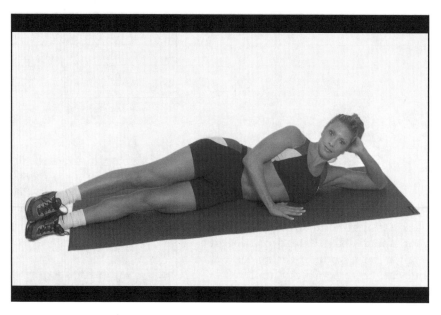

Start/Finish:
Lie on your side with
your body straight.

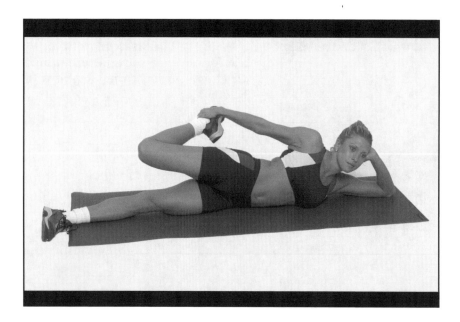

The Stretch:
Bend your top leg at the
knee and grasp your
foot with your hand just
below the ankle. Pull
the leg back with your
hand and feel a mild
stretch. Repeat with the
other leg.

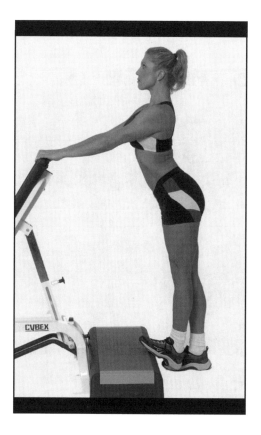

THE
CALVES

Standing
Calf
Stretch

Start/Finish:
Stand on a step or raised surface with the ball of one foot.

The Stretch:
Lean forward and feel your calf and ankle stretching. There should be no tension or pulling feeling behind your knee.

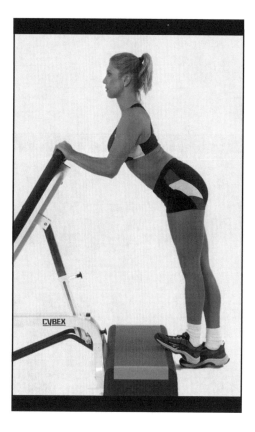

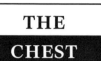

THE
CHEST

Standing Chest Stretch

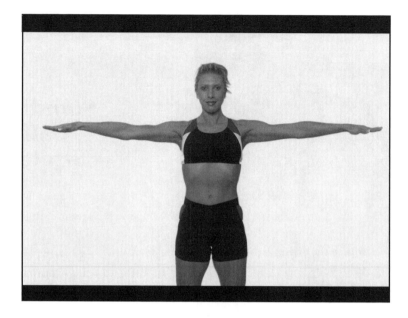

Start/Finish:
Stand up straight with your feet shoulder-width apart. Lift your arms out straight so that they form a "T" with palms down.

The Stretch:
Turn palms up while rotating thumbs backward. Stick out your chest at the same time you are pulling your arms backward. Bring your arms back to the starting position and repeat, stretching your arms back slightly further each time. Repeat five times.

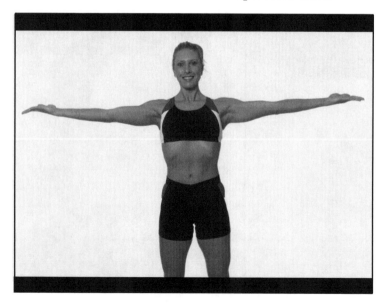

SHOULDERS & UPPER BODY

Standing Shoulder and Back Stretch

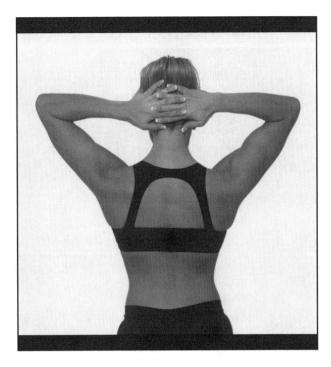

Start/Finish:
Interlace your fingers behind your head, holding your elbows straight out.

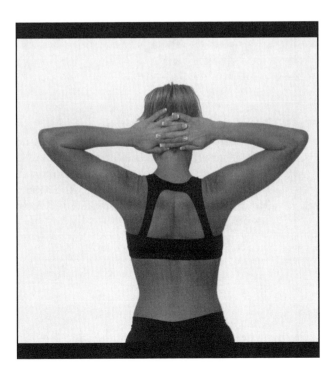

The Stretch:
Pull arms back and shoulder blades together and feel the stretch through your shoulders and upper back. Repeat slowly five times.

SHOULDERS & UPPER BODY

Shoulder, Triceps, and Side Stretch

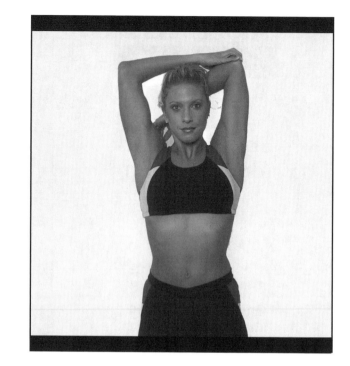

Start/Finish:
Place one arm overhead and bend it behind your head.

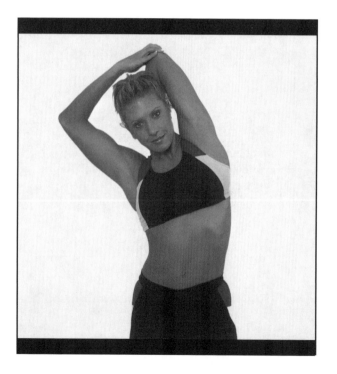

The Stretch:
Carefully pull your elbow further behind your head with your other arm as you slowly bend to one side. Feel the mild stretch in your triceps, shoulder, rib cage, and waist. Hold until the stretch is completed. Repeat on other side.

A Final Note on Stretching

Stretching can and should be a critical addition to your fitness program. A great deal of chronic pain that people feel, particularly as they age, is related to years of structural and musculature imbalances, particularly in the lower extremities. Shortened muscles that are not stretched can result in damage to the ligaments, which in turn contributes to bad posture and loss of strength and function. In addition, incorrect stretching can cause further damage. Make proper stretching a major part of your active fitness lifestyle and enjoy excellent health without pain.

—*Strength Training*—

Many people find the idea of strength training or bodybuilding intimidating. Questions like "where do I begin if I've never done this before" or "when will I find the time" are bound to come up. Actually, the most important question is whether you really want to change your lifestyle to be more fitness-oriented and so that you can enjoy all of the great benefits that go along with being fit. If you do, you will be able to work around the practical inconveniences to achieve your desired results. These inconveniences will seem much less important as your fitness lifestyle becomes a positive habit in your life.

What you may ultimately discover is that your fitness lifestyle causes positive changes in other areas of your life. For instance, if time is a limiting factor preventing you from exercising, consider an occupation where you can work from home (see Chapter 3, "The Home-Based Business Revolution") and avoid the waste of time and the hassle associated with commuting. Consider everything and anything that is preventing you from looking and feeling better. After all, when you look and feel your best, you are more capable of being a positive influence on others. Strength training can lead to many other marvelous changes in your life that you may never have considered before. Consider them now!

One of the first questions to answer when embarking on your quest for a "better body" is to determine where to work out. I have always preferred the combination of a home gym with membership at a health club. I like this approach because sometimes it is just more convenient to work out at home and avoid the traffic and save time. However, the variety of weight-training equipment found in health clubs today would be very expensive to duplicate at home even if you had a large enough home to put it in. There is, of course, the added consideration of preference. For some, the excitement and energy of the gym is a motivating factor to getting a good workout. For others, the privacy of working out at home is more appealing. I prefer the benefits of having both locations at my disposal.

The Home Gym

You may be surprised at how much you can accomplish at home with a minimal amount of equipment and cost. The choices we have today regarding home gym equipment and systems are many. You see them advertised on TV infomercials, in fitness magazines, and on the Internet. I find most of the exercise equipment advertised completely unnecessary, regardless of the cost. As with many other things in life, when it comes to fitness equipment, simple is best. You can get an excellent workout at home with the following pieces of basic exercise equipment:

- *A set of dumbbells.* The weights you select will be dependent on your strength level, but in a short time you will know what weights suit you best. If used properly, dumbbells provide you with the ability to perform a wide variety of exercises, develop an excellent range of motion, and enable you to have a safe workout.

- *A good sturdy weight bench.* A basic weight bench with an adjustable back to allow varying degrees of incline will allow you to perform many types of weight training exercises. In general, the wider the cushions on the bench and "footprint" of the bench, the better support your body will get. Get the best one you can afford. A good one will last many years with a minimal amount of care. As you gain experience, you will notice and appreciate a good workout bench.

- *A dumbbell rack.* You can find a good-quality dumbbell rack at a reasonable price. It's really nice to able to place the dumbbells somewhere other than the floor, and it's much easier on your back and joints over time.

- *A good pair of weight-training gloves.* I prefer the ones with velcro wrist support. Gloves will give you a better grip, save your hands from a lot of wear and tear, and reduce the chance of injury. I can't tell you how many times weight-training gloves have saved my hands from cuts, bruises, and, quite possibly, more serious injury.

Home Gym Guidelines

Working out at home is a much different experience from working out at the gym. You are in control of the environment, so use it to your advantage. Here are some tips:

- One of the best ways to enhance your workouts at home is to play the type of music you enjoy, music that gets you motivated and inspired. Whatever that type of music is, play it and experience the difference.

- Establish a workout ritual. Having some form of workout regimen will get you in the mood and keep you there. A workout ritual could be as simple as your warm-up routine or the sequence of music you listen to. There's something about merely putting on my workout gloves that signals to my brain that I'm ready to "get it on" with my workout. Find a ritual that makes you feel this way.

- Your workout time is your time for yourself, but if you have a serious workout partner at home, that's great! However, once your workout has begun, any distraction will take away from its effectiveness. If you have family members at home, ask them not to disturb you; tell them that this is your "personal time." I suggest letting your voice mail answer the phones as well.

    Time is becoming an increasingly precious commodity as changes in society progress. *Don't allow people to waste your precious time.*

- Drink water even when you're not thirsty, and always have a water bottle next to you!

- Work out no more than one hour per session. If you are working out correctly—which at a pace that is not too hurried and not too slow, but working out with passion and intensity—one hour is plenty. I find that between 45 minutes and one hour is ideal. In addition, for best results work out three to six times per week. Never train any body part two days in a row; this advice applies whether you are working out at home or at the health club.

Health Club Workout Tips

Working out at the health club is a different experience from working out at home. However, getting a great workout should be your primary purpose regardless of the location. Here are a few tips for maximizing your workout at the gym:

- Do not be intimidated by the big bodybuilders. They weren't born looking that way, and most of them are concentrating on their workouts as you are. Feel at ease to use any piece of equipment you wish anywhere in the gym. Virtually any serious bodybuilder will respect someone who is putting forth great effort at the gym (as I'm sure you will be!).

- Bring a towel (and your water, of course).

- Don't be shy about asking for assistance if you need it. You'd be amazed at how many people at the gym are also first-time bodybuilders. Most experienced bodybuilders will be happy to help.

- Some people use the gym as an excuse to "hang out" with friends and waste time. Having friends and spending time with them is great, but you'll have to determine for yourself whether you want to hang out or work out at the gym. After a great workout, the time you spend with your friends will be much more enjoyable.

- Always be aware of other bodybuilders around you at the gym and what types of weights they may be lifting or carrying, particularly in the free-weight area. Safety should always be your number-one priority, so keep a safe distance between yourself and other weight-lifters.

- Don't ever try to impress anyone with how much weight you can lift. Weight training is not about how much weight you can lift but about what improvements you can make to your body. The weights are simply the tool that you are using; the actual weight of the tool is unimportant.

- Working out with a competent, compatible, and serious workout partner can be very beneficial, but finding someone who shares your busy schedule and commitment to a better body and lifestyle can be challenging.

- Use the auxiliary health club facilities to your advantage. Some clubs offer features such as pools, tanning beds, aerobics classes, juice bars, and child-care facilities.

Regardless of where you are working out, always use good weight-lifting form and technique. In addition, the old saying "no pain, no gain" went the way of the dinosaurs a long time ago. What you are looking for is progressive and consistent improvement through a gradual increase in the weights you lift, not some barbaric experience of testing how much pain you can withstand. Enjoy your weight-lifting opportunity, and always make it a positive and fun experience.

Your Strength Training Routine

In planning your exercise routine, work specific muscle groups or body parts on different days. You will therefore need multiple workout programs that will allow you to more effectively train and rest specific areas of your body. One common beginner's mistake is to work out the entire body at once; another is not having a well-thought-out plan.

Think of your body as having three main sections:

- Abdominal or midsection
- Lower body, including legs, hips, and gluteus maximus
- Upper body, including chest, arms, shoulders and back

Think of your upper body as divided into two subsections:

- Upper body front, including chest, biceps (front of upper arm), and shoulders (front and lateral deltoids)

- Upper body back, including your back, triceps (back of upper arm) and shoulder muscles (rear deltoids)

In addition, try to alternate between your lower body routine and upper body routine to give your body parts a chance to rest and grow. Remember, growth in muscle takes place during rest, not during exercise; but the exercise is necessary to produce the muscle growth. Also, it's a good idea not to have your aerobics day just before the day you are doing your lower-body strength training workout.

With all exercises, attempt to do 8–10 repetitions in each set. Do a total of four sets for each exercise. Gradually increase the weights for each set. For instance, during the first set of eight repetitions, you may only use a 10-pound pair of dumbbells. For the next set, you may feel comfortable progressing to a 15-pound pair, and so on. Your first set is always your warm-up set so always go light on this set with more repetitions.

Breathing is also extremely important. Exhale when pushing, pressing, or lifting the weights (positive movement), and inhale when lowering the weight (negative movement). *Never hold your breath!*

Motivation

I hear many different types of excuses regarding why people are unable to work out. Working out is your choice—something that only you can decide you will do or not do. I love to work out and need little extra motivation to head off to the gym or into my home gym.

However, if you want to experience a higher level of achievement, there is nothing like thinking of someone whose acts of bravery and courage inspire us to go beyond our limits. Actor Christopher Reeve (of *Rear Window,* the *Superman* movies, and many others) suffered a spinal cord injury in a 1995 equestrian accident. Reeve is determined to walk again, and I have no doubt that he will accomplish his objective. When I need motivation, I think of Christopher Reeve.

Dumbbell Squats

Gluteus Maximus and Thighs

Strength Training Exercises

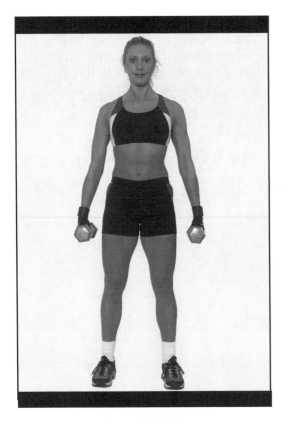

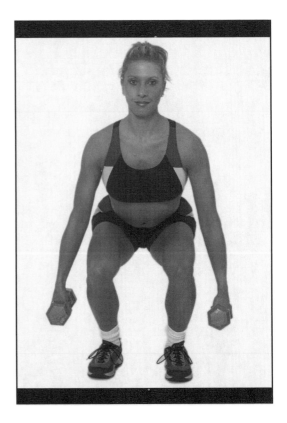

LOWER BODY
WORKOUT

The largest muscles in your body are in the lower extremities, so this is the best place to start. In any of your workouts, work the largest muscle groups first. Here are some very effective lower-body strength training routines:

Start/Finish:
Begin in an upright position with dumbbells at your sides. Face your palms in with your feet shoulder-width apart, and look straight ahead of you.

The Movement:
Bend your legs and lower your body so that your upper legs are parallel with the floor. Keep your back as straight as possible, and continue looking forward. Rise back up to the starting position.

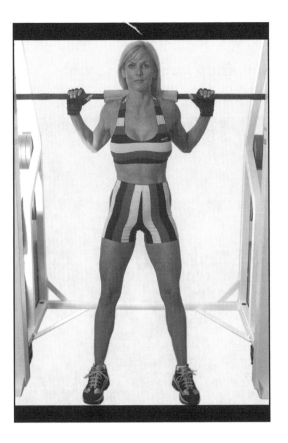

Smith Machine Squats

Gluteus Maximus and Thighs

Start/Finish:
Position yourself at the midway point underneath the bar. Place your feet shoulder-width apart and look straight ahead.

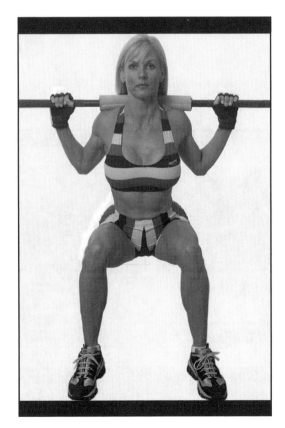

The Movement:
Raise up the bar by extending your legs, releasing the safety latches on the machine. Now lower yourself to where your upper legs are parallel to the floor. Push up with your legs and buttocks to an upright position.

The advantages of Smith Machine squats are that there is a safety latch attached to the bar and that there is support from the guides on the machine. In spite of these advantages over other forms of squat routines, always maintain proper form and use the same degree of caution as you would with any strength-training movement.

LOWER BODY
WORKOUT

Leg Press
Gluteus Maximus and Thighs

Start/Finish:
Position your feet shoulder-width apart and in the center of the footplate. Release the safety latches with your hands and push the weights up to the start position.

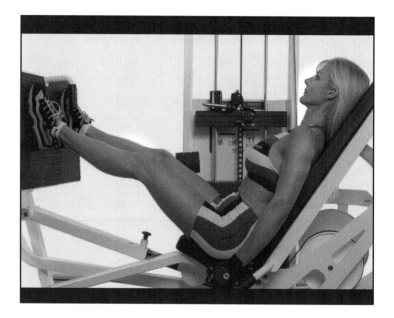

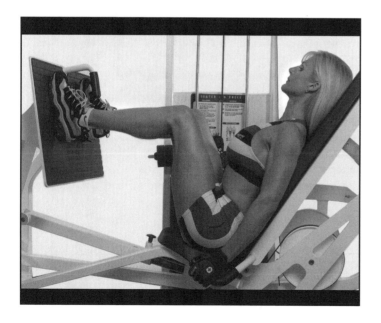

The Movement:
Lower the weight towards your chest until your hips begin to curl off the seat. Your lower back should be pressed against the seat back at all times. Push the weight back up to the starting position without locking your knees.

Lying Leg Curl

Hamstrings (backs of legs)

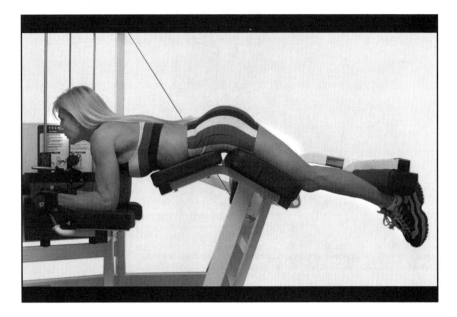

Start/Finish:
Lie face down on a leg-curl machine and grasp the handles lightly on the sides of the machine (do not cheat with your arms). Position the pads just above your ankles.

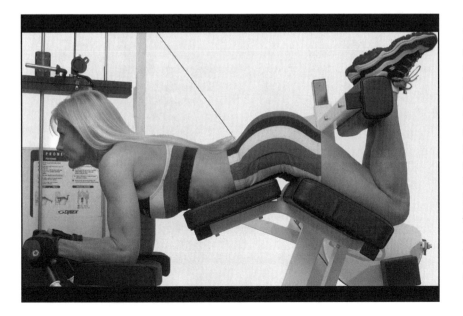

The Movement:
Raise your legs up as far as they will go, using the muscles of the upper backs of your legs. Contract your muscles at the maximum position and hold for one or two seconds. Return to the starting position at a controlled and moderate pace. To help avoid injuring your knees or lower back, do not lock your knees out or lift abdominals off the bench at any time.

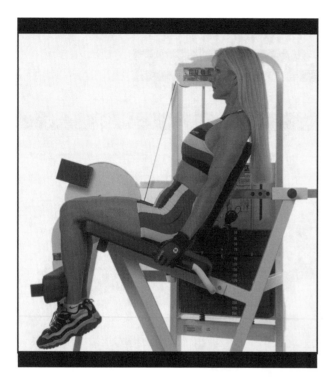

Leg Extension

Thighs

Start/Finish:

Adjust the seat back so that your back is supported and the footpads are just above your ankles.

The Movement:

Raise up your legs as far as they will go and squeeze your thighs at the maximum point. Lower your legs, but do not allow the weight stack to touch down. Use a full range of motion.

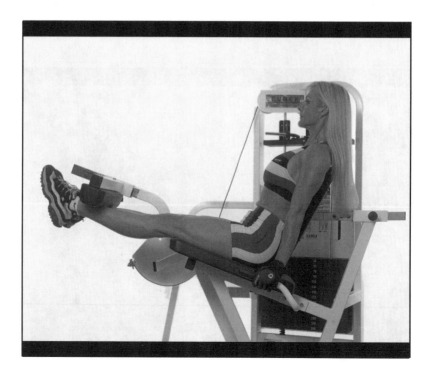

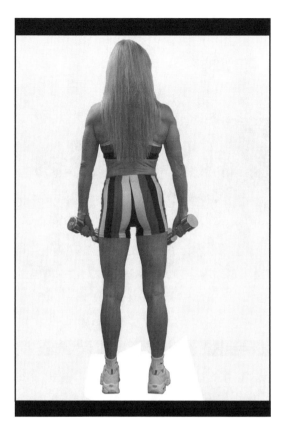

Dumbbell Calf Raises

Calves

This is one of the simplest calf exercises and my favorite.

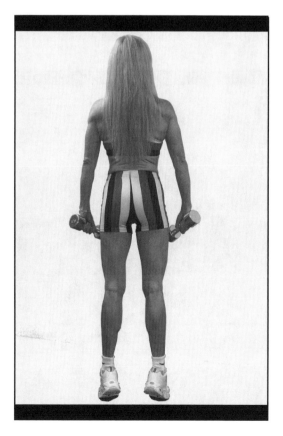

Start/Finish:
Stand with your feet flat on the floor with toes turned slightly outward.

The Movement:
While maintaining good posture with legs straight, raise yourself as high as you can on your toes. Hold and squeeze your calves at the top for a count of 2. Do four sets.

UPPER BODY
FRONT

Flat-Bench Dumbbell Press

Chest

Upper body front:
chest, biceps, shoulders

Start/Finish:
Lie face up on bench with your palms facing up and a dumbbell in each hand.

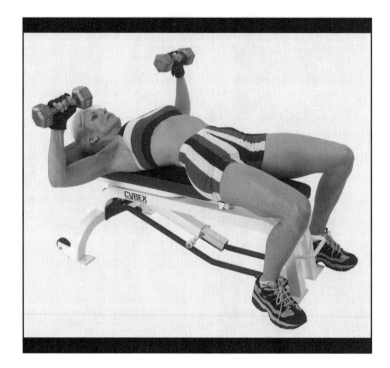

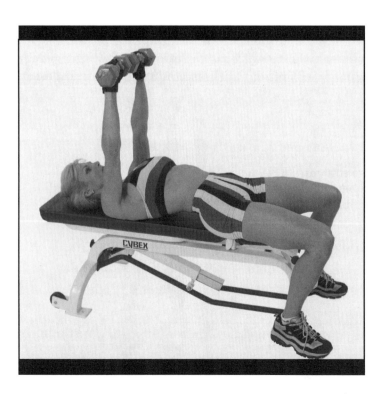

The Movement:
Raise the dumbbells straight up without touching them together to a point just before locking out your elbows. Lower the dumbbells to the start position.

Begin with light dumbbells until you feel comfortable balancing the weights.

UPPER BODY
FRONT

Incline Dumbbell Press

Chest and Shoulders

This exercise will also take some initial getting used to. Because of the angle, start with a lighter weight than you did with the flat dumbbell press.

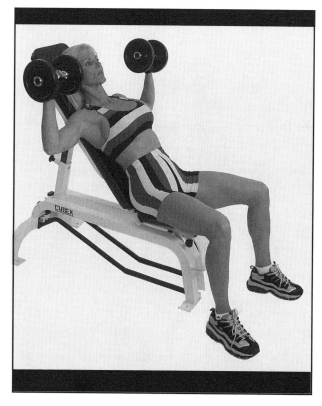

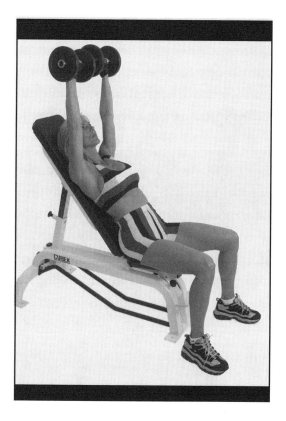

Start/Finish:
Perform this similarly to the flat-bench dumbbell press.

The Movement:
Press the dumbbells in an arc motion over the top of your chest, palms facing forward. Lower the weights slowly to the starting position.

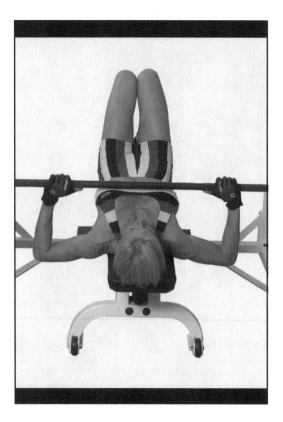

Smith Machine Decline Bench Press
Chest

I prefer using the Smith Machine when doing decline presses because using dumbbells on a decline bench is very awkward when picking up or lowering the dumbbells to the floor.

Start/Finish:
Position yourself so that the bar comes just above your lower chest at the bottom of the movement and keep your elbows pointed outward.

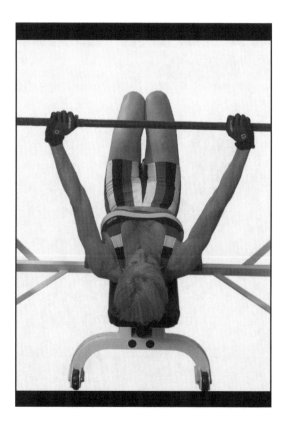

The Movement:
Push the weight bar up just before locking elbows. Lower to the point where your upper arms are parallel to the floor.

UPPER BODY
FRONT

Flat Bench Flyes

Chest

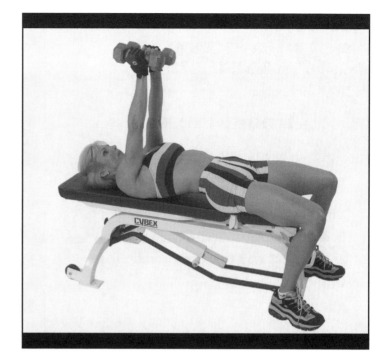

Start/Finish:
Lie on a flat bench with a dumbbell in each hand over your chest. Extend your arms with palms facing in.

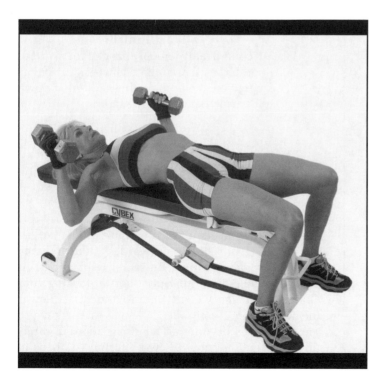

The Movement:
Lower the dumbbells to your sides in an arc motion with elbows partially bent. Your hands should be approximately parallel to your chest. (Do not go too low as this can damage your shoulder joint.) Raise dumbbells in an arc motion to the starting position.

UPPER BODY
FRONT

Arnold Press

Shoulders

This movement, named after famous bodybuilder Arnold Schwarzenegger, is an excellent way to work virtually the entire shoulder area.

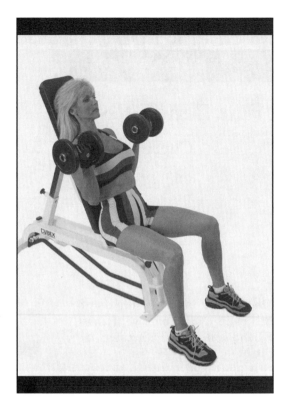

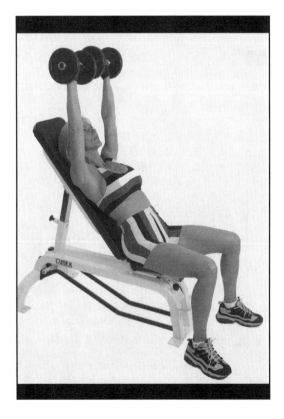

Start/Finish:

Sit comfortably on the bench, feet on the floor. Grasp the dumbbells with your palms facing your body and elbows pointed down with arms bent to your side.

The Movement:

Press the dumbbells upward and, as you do so, begin turning your hands outward. At the halfway point your palms should be facing each other. At the top, extend arms fully just short of locking your elbows, with the weights almost touching. Lower the weights in a controlled manner as you reverse the dumbbells by rotating hands in opposite direction. Your palms should now be facing you back at the starting position.

UPPER BODY

FRONT

Standing Dumbbell Lateral Raise

Shoulders

Start/Finish:

Stand straight up with dumbbells in hands and arms slightly bent at the elbows.

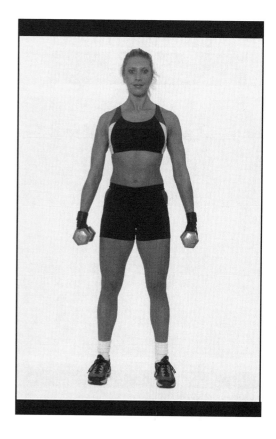

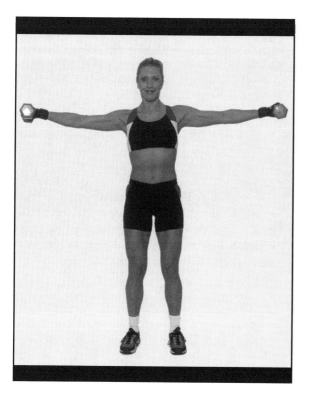

The Movement:

Raise the dumbbells out to the sides until your arms are parallel to the floor, keeping your palms facing down. After "squeezing" at the top, return to the starting point.

Resist the temptation to use "body English" to jerk the weights up. If you find yourself doing this, reduce the weights you are using.

UPPER BODY
FRONT

Seated Dumbbell Press

Shoulders

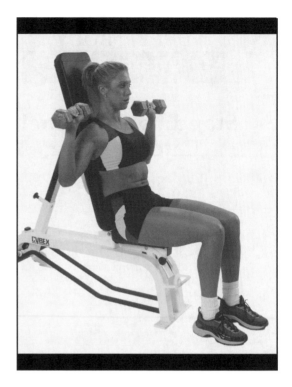

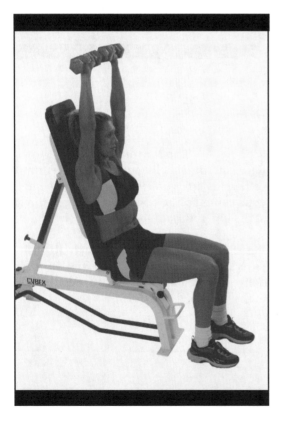

Start/Finish:
Sit upright on the bench with your back supported, grasping the dumbbells with your palms forward, elbows out.

The Movement:
Press the dumbbells overhead with an arcing motion just short of locking elbows. Lower the weights in a controlled fashion. Keep your torso straight throughout the movement.

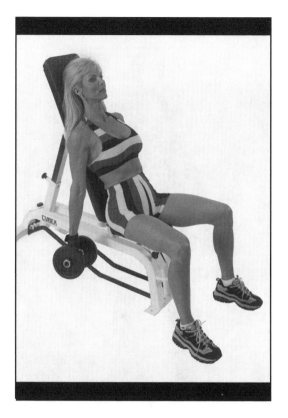

Seated Incline Dumbbell Curl

Biceps

Using the bench in an inclined angle allows you to work your biceps from a more beneficial "stretched" position.

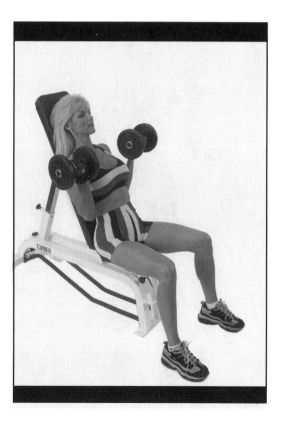

Start/Finish:

Grasp a pair of dumbbells palms-up while seated on an incline bench. Keep shoulders back and pressed against the pad. Keep your elbows in a stationary position with dumbbells at your side.

The Movement:

Lift the dumbbells as far as you can and squeeze your biceps briefly at the top. Return to the start position. As you increase the weights on this movement, you may find it more beneficial to alternate lifting the dumbbells one arm at a time.

UPPER BODY
FRONT

Dumbbell
Hammer Curl

Biceps

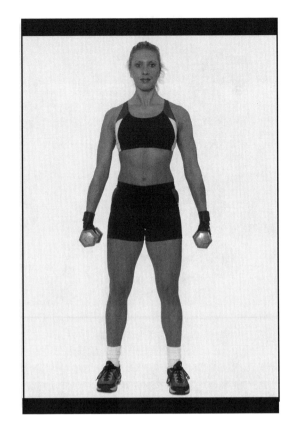

Start/Finish:
Stand up straight facing forward. Grasp dumbbells at your side, palms facing in.

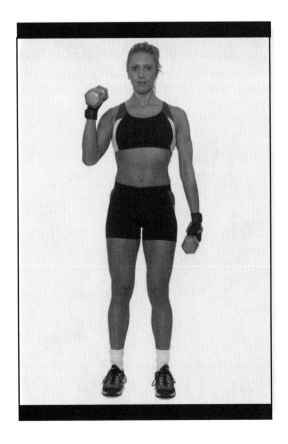

The Movement:
Curl one dumbbell up towards your front shoulder and squeeze briefly. Lower the dumbbell to your side and repeat with the other arm.

If you find yourself using your back to assist, the weight is too heavy; try some lighter dumbbells.

UPPER BODY
BACK

Dumbbell Rows

Upper body back:
back, triceps, and
shoulders
(rear deltoids)

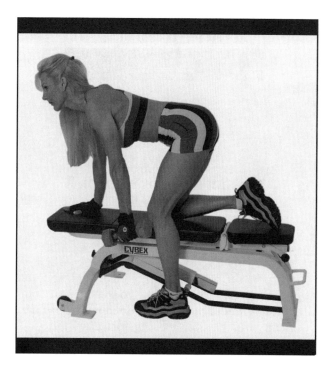

Start/Finish:
Place one knee on the bench with one foot flat on the floor. Place one hand on the bench (same side as knee on bench). Be sure to keep your back straight and eyes facing forward. Do not arch your back or let your head drop down.

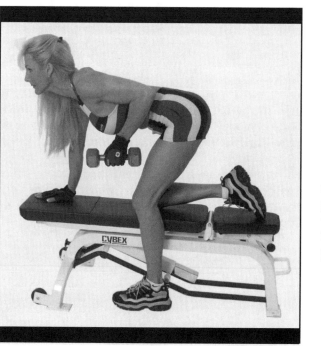

The Movement:
Grasp one dumbbell with the opposite hand, palm facing in. Lift the dumbbell as far as it will go, your upper arm being almost parallel with your body. Lower the weight. Repeat with other side.

UPPER BODY
BACK

Lat Pulldown

Latissimus Dorsi
(sides of upper back
and upper back)

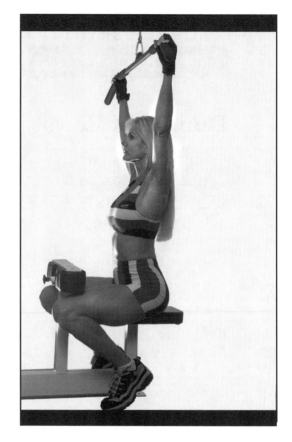

Start/Finish:
Sit up straight on a lat pulldown machine and adjust the seat pad so that your thighs fit comfortably under the leg pad. Keep your torso and head straight, eyes looking forward.

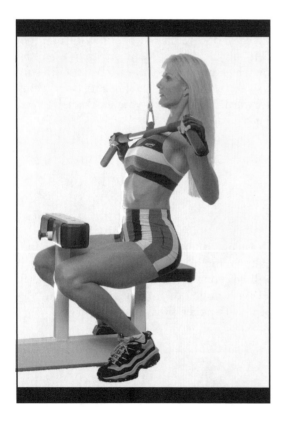

The Movement:
Grasp the bar with a wide grip and pull it down to just under your chin, in the upper chest area. Hold briefly and return to the top.

If you are using a weight that is too heavy, there will be a tendency to jerk the weights down. Concentrate on using your back muscles as much as possible.

UPPER BODY
BACK

This is a great back exercise
if your gym has the machine.

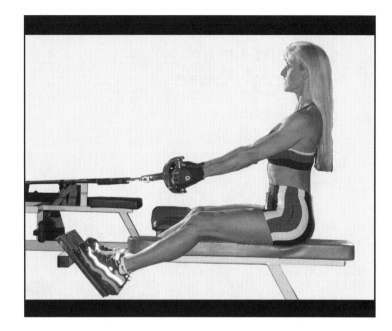

Seated
Cable Rows

Back

Start/Finish:
Sit on the pad with
your feet flat on the
footpad.

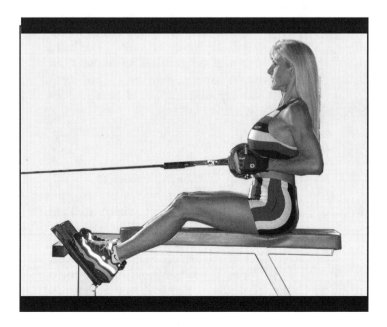

The Movement:
Grab the double-grip bar
and, in a smooth motion,
pull it back into the area
of your upper midsec-
tion. Keep your head up,
eyes forward, and back
straight. Concentrate on
using your back, not your
legs, and do not bend
forward at the waist.

UPPER BODY
BACK

Bent-Over
Lateral Raise

Shoulders
(rear deltoids)

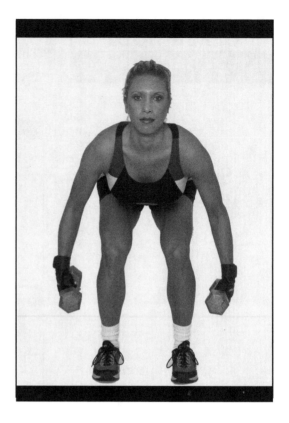

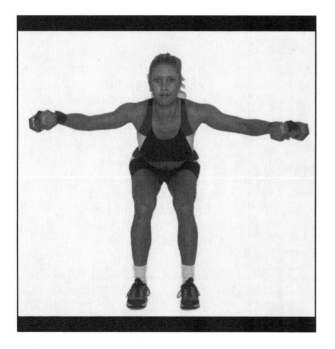

Start/Finish:
Hold a pair of dumbbells and bend over at the waist, back straight and eyes looking forward. Your back should be parallel with the floor, your arms should be slightly bent, and your feet should be shoulder-width apart.

The Movement:
Raise the dumbbells out to your sides, to the point where your upper arms are parallel with your back. Squeeze at the top and return to the start position. Always keep your knees bent and back straight, and do not look down as this will tend to make you hunch your back.

UPPER BODY
BACK

Dumbbell Kickback

Triceps
(back of upper arm)

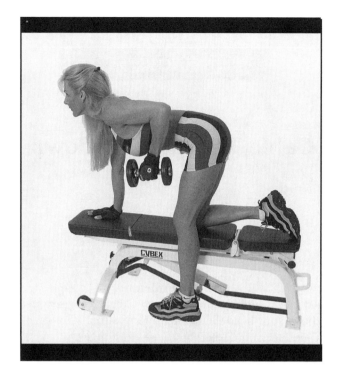

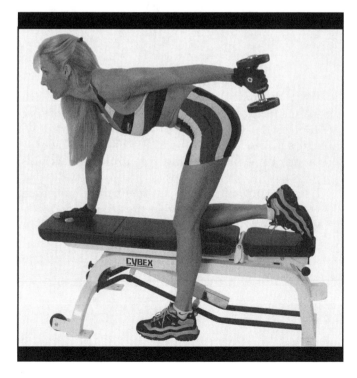

Start/Finish:
Place one knee on the bench and put your hand on it as well for support. Keep that arm straight. Hold a dumbbell with the other hand, palm facing in. Bend your arm so that your upper arm is parallel to your body.

The Movement:
Push the weight back, keeping your elbow in a stationary position, and squeeze your triceps at the top; then lower to the start position.

Avoid swinging the dumbbell as this exercise requires very strict form.

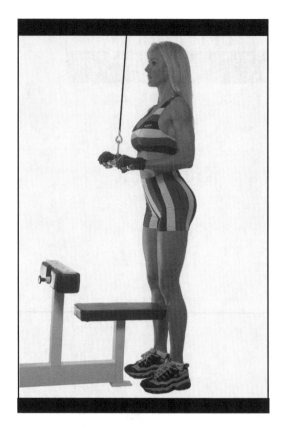

UPPER BODY

BACK

Cable Triceps Pressdown

Triceps

Start/Finish:

Attach a small straight bar to a cable pulley just above your head. Bend slightly forward at the waist. Your feet should be shoulder-width apart.

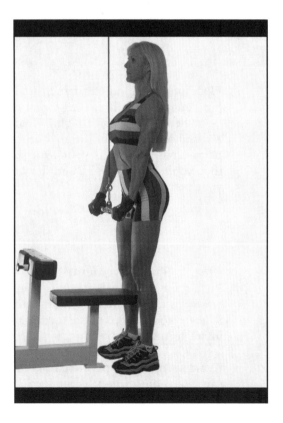

The Movement:

With the bar chest high, use an overhand grip (palms facing down) with your forearms almost parallel to the ground. Press the bar straight down and squeeze your triceps at the bottom. Slowly let the bar come back, staying in control of the weights.

Use a somewhat slower and deliberate movement with this exercise, and avoid the temptation to use your back or midsection to push the weight down.

ABDOMINALS
WORKOUT

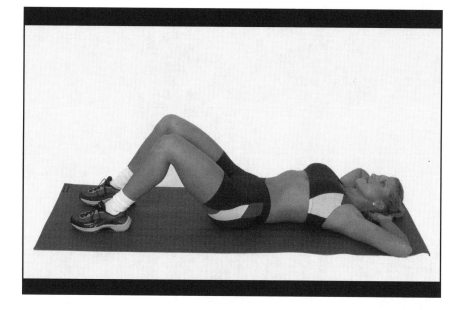

Basic Crunch

Start/Finish:
Lie on your back with your knees bent and feet flat on the floor. Support your head and neck with clasped hands, but do not use your hands to lift up as this will put pressure on your neck.

The Movement:
Slowly crunch your torso up, keeping your lower back pressed to the floor. Squeeze your abdominals briefly at the top. Lower your torso. Repeat ten times, and do four sets of ten repetitions.

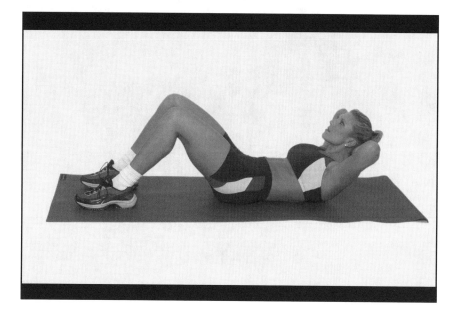

ABDOMINALS
WORKOUT

Decline sit-ups are challenging, but you will get good results if you do them correctly and put in the effort.

Decline Sit-ups

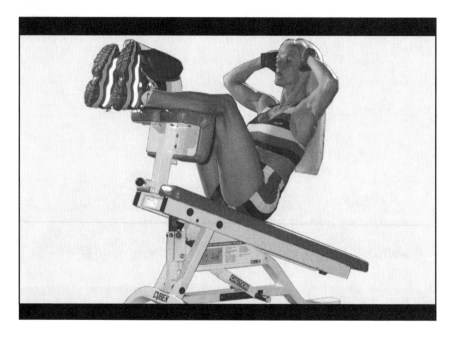

Start/Finish:
On a decline bench, fit your feet under the pads. Do not lie down on the bench, but remain in an upright sitting position. Place your fingertips by your temples, and do not clasp your hands behind your neck as this could stress your neck.

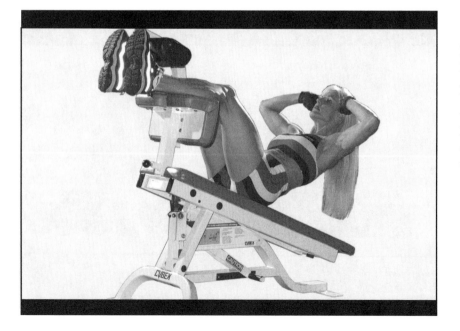

The Movement:
Lower your torso about halfway to the bench and squeeze your abs briefly. Come back up to the starting position. Repeat ten times, and do four sets of ten repetitions.

ABDOMINALS
WORKOUT

Side Crunches

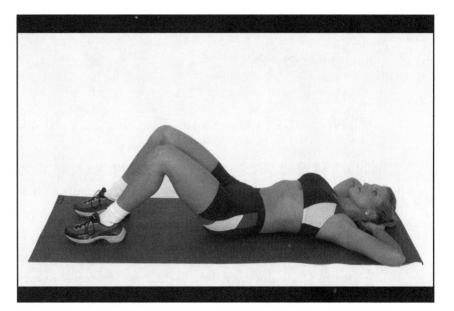

Start/Finish:
Lie on your back with your fingertips supporting your head and neck. Your elbows should be extended out to your sides.

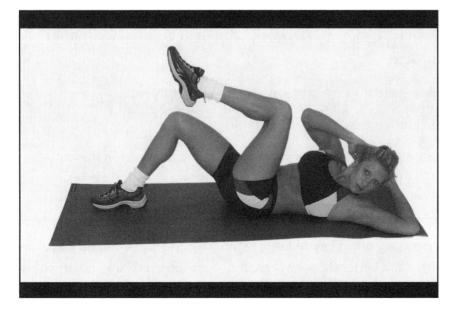

The Movement:
With your right foot on the floor, bend your right knee and extend your left leg. Start bending your left leg and move it towards your right shoulder. At the same time, move your right shoulder towards your left knee. Squeeze abdominals and hold the position for 1–2 seconds. Repeat fifteen times. Repeat on other side.

Putting It Altogether

As you begin your strength-training routine, it will be helpful to think of yourself as having four distinct but equally important body parts to train:

- Abdominals ("abs")

- Lower body—gluteus maximus, thighs, hamstrings, and calves

- Upper body—front: chest, shoulders (front and lateral deltoids), and biceps

- Upper body—back: back, shoulders (rear deltoids), and triceps

As much as most people dislike the idea of working abdominals, these muscles are absolutely crucial to your fitness success. The more you do them correctly and with proper form, the more results you will see. After a while you will look forward to your abdominal workout as you become accustomed to having a strong and shapely mid-section. That being said, it's still easy to leave the abdominal work for the end of your workout and then not have time to do them justice—or worse, forget them completely; I think we've all been guilty of this at one time or another. Here are some suggestions on how to prevent an unnecessary "battle of the bulge":

- Do your abdominals first thing in the morning. (I am not a morning person at all, but my abs are something I enjoy working on first thing before breakfast. I feel as if I have done something productive so it makes me feel good about my day from the start!)

- Use abdominals as part of your warm-ups before weight training.

- Incorporate abdominals into your aerobics workout.

- Leave plenty of time for abdominals if you are going to do them on the same day as your weight-lifting.

By the way, don't think that the fancy abdominal machines you see advertised are the magical solution or easy way out. They're not, I assure you. Basic abdominal exercises are at least as good as, if not better than, any machine-assisted exercises and probably safer as well.

In putting together your-weight training routine, include the weight-training exercises I have shown you how to do. I don't recommend doing them all on the same day. Alternating will give you the benefit of hitting your muscles in a slightly different way at different angles with each exercise.

Upper Body Workout Philosophy

You'll notice that the upper-body weight-training routines in the following pages have three variations:

- Upper body weight training—front

- Upper body weight training—back

- Upper body weight training—front and back

The reasoning behind this workout philosophy is that you can focus on one part of your upper body on different days. You can work on the front of your upper body or the back of your upper body, or combine both in an all-inclusive upper-body workout. Think of the all-inclusive workout as a "freestyle" day, on which you can work on virtually any upper body part you want. Spend the same amount of time and effort that day as you would on any workout day, paying particular attention to the areas you want to improve. Over the years I have been weight training, I have found that splitting your routines up in this fashion is a convenient and effective way to isolate the muscle groups of the upper body. And remember to always do your stretching after a light warm-up!

—*The Personal Touch*—
Designing Your Body-Specific Workout

One major drawback I see with most workout routines is that they do not take into consideration that each one of us is a unique person with a specific body type, metabolism rate, and varying responses to different forms of exercise. In order to get the most out of the time you devote to achieving the "better body" you want for yourself, it's important to follow a workout routine that will take best advantage of your athletic strengths and at the same time improve upon your weaknesses. Each of us is born with a particular genetic makeup; and while there is nothing you can do to change that, there's a tremendous amount you can do to improve upon what you were born with. First let's take a look at the three major body-type classifications—ectomorph, mesomorph, and endomorph—and the workout routines that will most benefit each body-type.

The Ectomorph

Ectomorphs tend to be tall and thin with a smaller, lighter bone structure. Ectomorphs also have relatively low levels of both body fat and muscle and a faster metabolism than other body-types.

Because of their lean build, ectomorphs tend to be good at aerobic exercises such as distance-running, cross-country skiing, fitness-walking, and other forms of high-endurance exercises. Most ectomorphs are also very flexible and tend to excel at stretching-related activities such as yoga, but they are less proficient in activities involving strength movements or sudden bursts of speed.

Because of your naturally thin body-style, you will benefit the most from weight-training exercises. Weight training will add both bone and muscle onto your frame and help to put all the right curves in all the right places. Ectomorphic women will benefit greatly from the emphasis on strength training because their smaller bone structure puts them at a higher risk for developing osteoporosis. In addition, both men and women will benefit from building more muscular definition. One great thing about being an ectomorph is that, with a good weight-training program, you will be able to attain a high degree of muscular definition.

Ectomorph Weekly Workout Routine

Monday:
Lower-body weight training
Gluteus maximus, thighs, hamstrings, and calves
Abdominals

Tuesday:
Upper-body weight training—front
Chest, shoulders (front and lateral deltoids), and biceps

Wednesday:
Aerobics / abdominals / stretching

Thursday:
Upper-body weight training—back
Back, shoulders (rear deltoids), and triceps

Friday:
Lower-body weight training
Gluteus maximus, thighs, hamstrings, and calves
Abdominals

Saturday:
Upper-body weight training—front and back
Chest, shoulders (all), biceps, back, and triceps

Sunday:
"Enjoy Your Body" Day

The Mesomorph

Mesomorphs are the people most frequently referred to as "natural athletes." They have a higher-than- average concentration of fast-twitch muscle fibers, meaning that the men have very muscular and powerful physiques and women have a much greater ability to increase muscle mass. Athletic prowess tends to come naturally for these folks; however, mesomorphs do have a tendency to gain weight.

Mesomorphs are generally good at weight training and most sports activities, especially those requiring strength and short bursts of energy. Mesomorphs are not so adept at endurance sports as ectomorphs and should be careful not to over-train any body part lest they end up looking out of proportion. Also, frequent stretching is a must to prevent pulled muscles and stiffness.

When it comes to working out, mesomorphs should use a combination approach. Aerobics, stretching, and abdominals should receive priority. However, weight training two or three days a week will help maintain muscle tone and definition as well as fast metabolism.

Mesomorph Weekly Workout Routine

Monday:	Aerobics / stretching / abdominals
Tuesday:	Lower-body weight training Gluteus maximus, thighs, hamstrings, and calves
Wednesday:	Aerobics / stretching / abdominals
Thursday:	Upper-body weight training—back Back, shoulders (rear deltoids), and triceps
Friday:	Aerobics / stretching / abdominals
Saturday:	Upper-body weight training—front Chest, shoulders (front and lateral deltoids), and biceps
Sunday:	"Enjoy Your Body" Day

The Endomorph

Endomorphs tend to be heavy-set with a large bone structure and a slow metabolism. Don't be fooled, however—endomorphs are naturally strong; the problem is that there's usually too much padding to see any muscle definition.

Endomorphs are generally better at activities that require strength than at activities requiring endurance and agility, such as long-distance running or jumping. Endomorphs must concentrate on increasing their metabolic rate to shed pounds and improve body shape and muscle tone. A variety of aerobics activities should be used—non-weight-bearing (cycling, rowing and swimming) as well as weight-bearing (running, treadmill and step machine). While aerobics training should be stressed, weight training with higher than normal repetitions, medium weights, and little rest between sets will also serve to increase metabolism and improve overall body shape.

Endomorph Weekly Workout Routine

Monday: Aerobics / abdominals / stretching

Tuesday: Lower-body weight training
            Gluteus maximus, thighs, hamstrings, and calves

Wednesday: Aerobics / abdominals / stretching

Thursday: Upper body weight-training—front and back
            Chest, shoulders (all), biceps, back, and triceps

Friday: Aerobics / abdominals / stretching

Saturday: Aerobics / abdominals / stretching

Sunday: "Enjoy Your Body" Day

Combination Body Types

In reality, most people don't fit perfectly into just one category of body type. Rather, most people are a combination of the three major body types but tend to favor one type over the others. For example, you may have a slim build (ectomorph) but also have the ability to build muscle (mesomorph); or you may have a tendency to be overweight (endomorph) but also have a very muscular frame (mesomorph). Use the body-specific workout routines as a guideline to your fitness training, and use the one that most closely fits your own unique body type. This will help you develop the body shape and reach the fitness goals you most desire in the least amount of time.

RECOMMENDED HEALTH AND FITNESS MAGAZINES

- *American Health & Fitness*
- *Health*
- *Men's Fitness*
- *Men's Health*
- *Ms. Fitness*
- *Muscle and Fitness*
- *MuscleFitness Hers*
- *Oxygen Fitness*
- *Shape*

On page 287 you will find a Daily Workout Log that you can customize for your special body building program.

Working out should be fun—and if you work on it consistently, you will begin to enjoy your new body! You worked hard for it and earned it, and you also get to walk around with it. You're going to look fabulous. Congratulations on making the effort to change into a better you!

DAILY WORKOUT LOG

DAY	DATE	MUSCLE GROUPS WORKED	EXERCISE	WT. USED (LBS.)	SET	REPS	NOTES

Conclusion

IT'S FUNNY how we remember things, but I'll never forget something one of my football coaches, Erwin Gerung, once said to me. One Monday afternoon, while watching game films, he said; "Anthony, whatever you do on the field or in life, always keep moving in a forward direction and don't look back, because moving forward will take you where you want to go. . . . " Those words have stuck with me to this day. In many ways, my wish for you is that *The Total Package* will inspire you to move forward with your life, on the journey to achieving your ultimate lifestyle. In the final analysis, the decision to achieve your ultimate lifestyle is your choice and your choice alone. True change—in this case, the change necessary to create your ultimate lifestyle—will take effort, but the rewards will probably be some of the most significant ones you will achieve in your lifetime.

The achievement of your own personal "ultimate lifestyle" will require that you focus on attaining a *balanced lifestyle,* which means having control over of all facets of your life including your finances and investments, nutrition, fitness, relationships, spiritual beliefs, career, and home life. Of course, technology has woven its way into virtually every area of our lives. On the Internet today for instance, you can make complete travel reservations and map your travel route, buy a new or used car, earn a college degree, conduct real estate transactions, buy a mortgage, and even find a date for

Saturday night! Embrace the Internet and other key technologies as tools to help you grow and enjoy life to the fullest. However, don't forget that technology is just one of the tools at your disposal. Technology is wonderful, but remember—computers can't replace personal relationships and the *human touch*.

The Total Package is designed to take you step by step through each of the key areas of your life and help you design the lifestyle that most appeals to you. Many people never achieve their ultimate lifestyle because they tend to focus on only one or a few key lifestyle areas. For instance, many in our society have the false notion that achieving great wealth—or "getting rich" will lead to a lifetime of happiness. While having money is one part of achieving your ultimate lifestyle, large sums of money do not guarantee happiness. In fact, because of their lack of balance due to an overabundance of money and a concentrated focus on their wealth, many wealthy people actually sabotage their ability to attain an optimum lifestyle filled with happiness, excitement, and positive expectations. Other examples of people with unbalanced lifestyles include those who spend most of their lives trying to be the person someone else wants them to be; some become workaholics (or alcoholics), and others wait all week for the weekend to finally *have fun*. If having fun is important to you (and I hope it is), why not design your life so that you can have fun on Tuesday morning at ten o'clock? Why wait until the weekend? If you truly have balance, you will find yourself having fun much more of the time in one way or another. Without balance, true fulfillment in your life will be forever elusive. The key is balance; when you are out of balance in your life, it is difficult to achieve or enjoy true success. Remember as well that taking responsibility for your actions is part of being in balance. Never blame others for your own shortcomings; it's a waste of time and energy. Focus instead on learning from the experience and improving yourself in that area.

You now have the information you'll need to embark on your fantastic voyage to a life filled with infinite possibilities and joy that may be unimaginable to you right now. Regardless of your current circumstances, you have it inside of you to begin, to take at least one small step in the direction of your ultimate lifestyle. Do not be overwhelmed or intimidated by this thought in any way. Fear is an illusion you instantaneously create in your mind, and therefore you have the ability to dispel it just as quickly. Focus on what's ahead of you and not what you are leaving behind. If you concentrate your thoughts on moving forward and in the direction of your dreams, you will move in that direction. You can do it if you will just go one step at a time.

Use the principles and information I have provided you in *The Total Package* to your utmost advantage. Incorporate balance into your life, and experience the fulfilling life you deserve. Strive to create the ultimate *balanced* lifestyle for yourself and seek to make a positive difference in other people's lives. Build your life on a strong foundation and accept only win-win solutions and relationships. Have fun and cherish the many new, exciting and uplifting friends you'll meet along the way.

Congratulations on taking that critical first step, and never forget that you will always succeed if you get up one more time than you fall.

Anthony Palmer

For more information on success-building and health and fitness programs, visit

www.AnthonyPalmer.net

About the author

ANTHONY PALMER is dedicated to providing the education, inspiration, and resources to help people make lasting and positive changes in their lives.

He has a BBA from Florida Atlantic University's School of Business in Boca Raton, Florida, and an MBA from the Wayne Huizenga School of Business and Entrepreneurship at Nova Southeastern University in Fort Lauderdale, Florida. He began his financial planning career at American Express Financial Advisors and moved on to form his own firm in 1995. He holds the Chartered Mutual Fund Counselor^{SM} and Certified Annuity Advisor^{SM} professional designations.

An athlete who realized the many benefits of bodybuilding, he has conducted extensive research on nutrition, longevity, and the mind–body connection for over two decades. He is CEO and co-founder of a firm specializing in fitness, nutrition, anti-aging, and lifestyle development.

Anthony Palmer's companies offer

- *"Create Your Ultimate Lifestyle"* live events
- Lifestyle, career, and home-based business coaching
- Goal-setting and personal success plans
- Fitness, nutrition, and weight management programs
- All-natural anti-aging and health-care formulations

For more information on Anthony Palmer and his companies, visit his Web site:

www.AnthonyPalmer.net

Order *The Total Package*

by Anthony Palmer

Hardcover, 304 pages, illustrated, on permanent paper

ISBN 0-9744453-0-4

USA: *$25.00 per copy*   **CANADA:** *$35.95 per copy*

Shipping/handling: *USA $4.95, International $9.95*

Ship to:

Name: _____

Address:_____

_____

City_____State____Zip_____

Telephone number: (____) _____

Number of copies _____ x $_____ = _____

Add shipping/handling = _____

Add state sales tax (%) = _____

TOTAL _____

Method of payment: ❏ Check ❏ Money order

❏ Visa ❏ MasterCard ❏ Discover ❏ American Express

Card number _____ Exp. date_____

Name on card: _____

Cardholder's signature:

_____

Send payment with completed order form to:

Castiglione Publishing, Inc.
c/o Bookmasters, 30 Amberwood Parkway, Ashland, OH 44805
Tel: 1-800-247-6553 • Fax: 1-419-281-6883

www.AnthonyPalmer.net